Loving Deeds For The Children

A Man Called Hawk

Ron "Kwiet Storm" Smith

*Forewords by Antonio M. Yaniz, M.D.
and Thomas Kelly, Psy.D.*

iUniverse, Inc.
New York   Bloomington

Loving Deeds for the Children

A Man Called Hawk

iUniverse books may be ordered through booksellers or by contacting:

iUniverse
1663 Liberty Drive
Bloomington, IN 47403
www.iuniverse.com
1-800-Authors (1-800-288-4677)

ISBN: 978-1-4401-0489-3 (pbk)
ISBN: 978-1-4401-0490-9 (ebk)

Printed in the United States of America

iUniverse Rev. Date 10/28/08

Foreword

by
Antonio M. Yaniz, M.D.
Board Certified Psychiatrist

I have worked for 30 years with adolescents who have severe emotional and behavioral problems. I was the founder and director of an adolescent treatment program that included inpatient/outpatient, and partial hospitalization programs. I have been the psychiatrist in charge of the treatment plans in two large residential facilities for adolescents with behavioral problems and sexual offending behaviors for 14 years. In spite of my experience and accumulated knowledge, this book gave me new insights into the pathology of these adolescents and their treatment needs.

I have known Ronald Smith for many years, and I have witnessed how he works with the most dysfunctional and wounded adolescents that I have ever seen. I know that his high rate of success is due to his deep spirituality that makes him confident and his profound knowledge of adolescent dynamics. In this book, the reader will understand these qualities that the writer possesses.

Once you start reading this novel, it is very difficult to put down, and if you have ever been in contact with emotionally disturbed adolescents, this book will surprise you with a tremendous insight into the causes and the solutions for their issues.

Ronald Smith's literary style makes reading very easy and the elegance of his narration is delightful. I strongly recommend this book to parents, teachers, mental health workers, and even adolescents.

Foreword

by
Thomas Kelly, Psy.D.
Psychotherapist

Awe-inspiring.

Ron 'Kwiet Storm' Smith once again finds the passion and purpose in his characters that leave the reader feeling like making a difference. Drawing from his own many years of experience working with troubled and challenging – read fountains of opportunity – youth in residential treatment, Smith represents with passion, poetry, and grittiness the experiences of youth gone astray, as well as those special adults with the calling to help them find their way. The range of emotions and unique experiences of his characters in this pursuit of growth, healing, and self-discovery should ring real and true for anyone who has experienced the residential treatment of youth. Treatment providers, parents, youth on the brink of adulthood, or anyone invested in growing themselves by helping others to grow will instantly identify with the characters.

Although a novel, the parallel process of self-growth as a 'receiver' of treatment and as a 'provider' of treatment has rarely been so richly and personally presented. An intensely moving account of empathy, hope, and opportunity amidst the turbulence of youth without direction or guidance - youth without anyone to believe in them or recognize the vastness of their opportunities and potential.

Chapter 1
Lake Apache Academy
(The Yellow Phase)

It was a cool morning on the campus of Lake Apache. It was late August and the sun was just starting to rise above the eastern horizon. Dew settled on the freshly cut lawn. Senior Therapeutic Youth Counselor Horus Orion Hawkinson, a.k.a. Hawk, as his colleagues called him, stood on the lawn of an open grass field absorbing the rays of the rising radiant orb. He was wearing a Lake Apache t-shirt with matching sweat pants.

The physically fit, keen eyed, no nonsense disciplinarian and several of his colleagues including Ms. Maya Sunflower and Mr. Jimmy Minnis had just finished taking a physical performance test. They stood sharing small talk while waiting for the Lake Apache busses to arrive. The sight of the team standing together exemplified unity.

In the distance behind Hawkinson and his colleagues were the edifices of Lake Apache Academy. There was a large sporting complex, male youth dorms, female youth dorms, male staff sleeping quarters, female staff sleeping quarters, a business office, school, vocational center and a cafeteria. In the distance behind the sporting complex was an all weather track. Beyond the track was the beautiful, clear Lake Apache.

It was the dawn of a new day and a new cycle. Hawkinson had just completed his tenth cycle a month earlier. He was prepared mentally, spiritually and physically to begin his eleventh cycle on unit eight, which was the older adolescent male program. There were eight total units; four boy units and four girls.

Outside of being a youth counselor, Hawkinson served as a diversity trainer for his colleagues, a mentor for struggling teens, a volunteer basketball coach for children and a member of council for a school in his community. He was one active soul.

Each cycle at Lake Apache Academy lasted eleven months from late August until mid July. At the end of every cycle, the youth who completed the therapeutic treatment program were eligible to graduate. The graduates moved on to face the challenges and choices of a new reality. Some moved on to live with their legal guardians, while others ventured off to independent living programs or privately funded group homes.

Those that did not graduate earned the title "holdovers". The holdovers were recycled and given another chance to succeed at Lake Apache during the next cycle. The holdovers attended a late summer intensive treatment program for four weeks. It was to help prepare them for the up and coming cycle. If the holdovers did not succeed during the next cycle, some found themselves placed in a more restrictive environment.

After graduation, many of the staff who didn't work the summer holdover program took four to five weeks off to charge their batteries before the next cycle began. During the early cycles of his career, Hawkinson was one of those staff members who stayed over to work diligently with the holdovers. Just within the past couple of cycles, Hawkinson began taking the full five weeks off to recharge his batteries. The counselor was an advocate of self-care. It was a major key to his mental and spiritual health. Hawkinson took care of himself, which gave him the inner strength to take care of others.

Three Lake Apache charter busses carrying youth from all over the country pulled up in front of the academy. The youth stepped off the busses with garbage bags, duffle bags and worn luggage. Many wore huge afros or looked like hippies. A couple of the youth even had the 1980's mullet hairstyle.

The youth stood on the lawn before Hawkinson and his comrades and studied their new surroundings, especially the fourteen foot bronze Apache warrior statue. The statue resembled a man wearing a hawk headdress and stood on a 6'x6' concrete platform in the circle drive of the campus entrance. Many of the youth were amazed by the statue. By the distant look in the youths' eyes, Hawkinson concluded that most of them carried more baggage than they were unloading from the busses. It was angry, emotionally disturbed, spiritually deflated and mentally challenged types of baggage that darkened their spiritual auras.

Prior to the youth arriving, Hawkinson and his peers did their homework. They studied the youths' files the way pro-football players study their playbooks. The files described various crimes committed by the young men;

armed robbery, burglary, criminal damage to property, mob action, sexual misconduct and drug trafficking to name a few.

The goals for the youth during their stay at the academy would be to learn and internalize the cycles of their behaviors, self-discipline, social adequacy and self esteem. The program was designed to groom the youth into model citizens with attainable goals.

*   *   *   *   *

After role call and an introduction to the staff, Hawkinson, Sunflower and their colleagues prepared the youth for a rigorous round of calisthenics. Being in physical shape was a priority for the staff at Lake Apache. That's where the physical performance test (PPT) came into play. Sunflower and Hawkinson were similar in many ways. Both of them were highly energetic and physically fit individuals. They trained diligently every morning before work. Sunflower was an over the top fireball full of desire, motivation and passion which made her quite successful in many areas of her life. Hawkinson was a humble, passionate and motivated innovator who did not comprehend mediocrity. He had a bowl of ambition every morning followed by a tall glass of persistence.

When Sunflower first arrived on the campus as a rookie youth counselor, Hawkinson was appointed as her mentor. He led by example. He taught her to harness and mold her fiery passion into greatness and leadership. He also taught her that her job duty was not to save the youth from their many issues, which was something he learned early on in his career. The responsibility of a youth counselor was to guide the youth and teach them how to manage their many issues without personally taking on their issues. Hawkinson kenw the practitioner's number one rule in the counseling field— believe in the therapeutic application he or she is providing and never take any of the client's issues personally.

Hawkinson had many positive quotes that he fed daily to the youth. One of his favorites was, *The sun is always shining, even when the skies are sometimes gray.* To Hawkinson the sun symbolized happy positive feelings while the gloomy gray clouds symbolized unhappy negative feelings. Even though the sun can't be detected with the visible eye when behind the clouds, it is still shining brightly, one only has to believe.

Over the many cycles, Hawkinson observed a great deal of his colleagues exhaust all of their emotional strength, which meant they were suffering from the burnout syndrome. The average length of employment for a youth counselor at Lake Apache was one cycle. Hawkinson was on his eleventh. His philosophy for success was free flow, which meant he didn't take things personally, because it is what it is. He free flowed effortlessly. He felt that when one tries too hard, they fail hard. Consistency, free flow and positive thinking were the three key ingredients to his longevity and success at Lake Apache.

* * * * *

The youth stretched before the calisthenics work out. The purpose of the work out was to motivate the youth for the emotionally, mentally, physically and spiritually tough times that lay ahead. After the calisthenics, Hawkinson and his colleagues ran the youth around the all weather track. They ran the Indian run which meant the very last person in line sprinted past everyone to the beginning of the line and took over with a nice steady pace. This went on until everyone had a chance to lead.

Most of the youth complained and cursed the staff under their breath. Some of the smokers and alcohol abusers struggled as they sweated the toxins out of their systems. There were the few youth who did not complain or give up. They were the ones Hawkinson watched closely. History proved their type to be future leaders at Lake Apache.

After the heart pounding, muscle aching workout, Hawkinson and his team of colleagues lined the youth up and marched them beyond the track to sit around Lake Apache and cool off. The youth spread out and some sat in the grass. The exhausted ones hung their heads and panted heavily while the smokers and drug abusers ventured over to the tree line to vomit.

* * * * *

After sitting by the lake to cool off, the youth were marched in columns of two to the male dorms. As they entered the building, the youth were amazed at their reflections on the highly polished floors. The chief administrator, Mr. Davidson, often expressed the axiom that a clean and healthy environment made for a clean and healthy attitude. He believed that the physical environment influenced the youths' perceptions of themselves.

Before Mr. Davidson came to Lake Apache seven cycles ago, the academy was average at best. A few months after his arrival, the academy underwent a complete makeover. The walls were freshly painted. The floors were retiled and polished to perfection on a daily basis. The grass received a weekly cutting. The groundskeepers removed the clutter from around the buildings and the attitudes of the youth and staff improved after their environment changed.

Mr. Davidson made it his business every morning to go from unit to unit and building to building, greeting every employee and youth by name. He had ambition, character, integrity and one heck of a memory. Mr. Davidson was a man of his word. If he said he was going to do something, it was as good as done. Hawkinson admired and respected the character of the optimistic leader.

The fresh smell of a clean environment penetrated the youths' nostrils as they walked the hallways. A large painting of an Apache warrior wearing a hawk mask and colorful headdress while holding a flagpole stared at them from an extended wall. It was the same warrior as the statue standing outdoors. The blue hawk-like eyes peering from behind the mask of the warrior seemed to stare right through the youth. Next to the warrior painting on the wall was a large sign that said, *Unit 8 Home of the Warriors*.

During the tour, some of the youth marveled at their new environment, but there were those who frowned and turned up their noses. Most of the youth came from a negative, hostile environment. Their past homes hosted cold concrete floors instead of highly polished tile and carpet like the floors at Lake Apache. The walls from their past were dirty and full of graffiti, instead of freshly painted walls with positive quotes in frames like the walls at Lake Apache. Their past sleeping arrangements usually involved overcrowded jail cells with flat mattresses, instead of single rooms with firm, padded mattresses like the ones at Lake Apache. The bathrooms where they came from had an ice cold, stainless steel toilet in a corner with no privacy. At Lake Apache, there were six private restrooms and each had a safety mirror, sink, single shower, dressing bench and porcelain toilet. Five youth were to alternate using a restroom as well as cleaning it.

During the tour, the youth eyed a computer room. Down the hallway was a game room with the latest video game system and video games. Next to the game room was a small kitchenette with appliances. Adjacent to the kitchen was a large ballroom with sturdy chairs set up in a horseshoe position. A podium sat in front of the room.

Behind the podium were three large flags on the wall. There was the American flag, Illinois flag and Lake Apache flag. Underneath the three flags were three large pennants. A yellow pennant represented the first phase of the treatment program which was the orientation, behavioral and physical fitness phase. The yellow phase lasted through the first four months of treatment. A red pennant represented the second phase, which was the emotional and mental phase. The second phase lasted the next four months. A blue pennant represented the third phase also known as the recovery phase, which focused on spiritual enlightenment, relapse prevention, victim apology sessions and giving back. The blue phase covered the last three months of treatment. Each phase hosted several written assignments.

Around the corner from the grand room were staff offices, cleaning closets and rooms used for individual and small group therapy sessions. After the tour, the youth turned in their personal belongings for inventory. Whatever was appropriate for the environment they kept in their possession, the rest went to a storage warehouse on campus.

Later, the youth went to their dorm rooms to make their beds and settle into their new environment before showers and haircuts. Inside their rooms they found a single bed, wardrobe closet, desk and their clothing attire for the next eleven months. It was an exciting time for some of the youth, but for most it was the beginning of a long, unbearable journey.

A few cycles ago, Hawkinson, Sunflower and some of the other counselors approached the Lake Apache Academy board of directors about administering a uniform. The purpose of the dress code was to instill pride and self-worth while maximizing focus, order and discipline. Having a dress code minimized racially motivated brotherhoods, violent gangs and other criminal organizations some of the youth brought to the academy from former environments. The uniform minimized some of the youth theft issues as well as eliminated the run risk. Many of the youth did not want to be seen on campus with the uniforms, let alone off campus.

Folded neatly on each bed were their everyday uniforms; three pairs of khaki pants and three rust colored polo shirts with *Lake Apache Academy* stitched in tan letters above the left breast. Next to the uniforms were two gray cotton sweatsuits with *Lake Apache Academy* in rust colored letters across the chest. On the back was the number eight. A pair of tan dress pants, a white dress shirt and a rust color tie lay on each bed as well. The dress clothing was needed for the Board of Elders ceremony.

Underneath each bed was a pair of sneakers, brown leather buckskin shoes and a pair of work boots. Inside the wardrobe was a rust colored fleece jacket with the Lake Apache warrior mascot sewn on the front left side. A winter coat, hat, gloves and pajamas hung in the wardrobe as well. At the bottom of the wardrobe was a plastic basket equipped with hygiene products.

Personal hygiene for most of the youth was an area that needed extra attention. It was at the top of Hawkinson's self-esteem list for the youth, right along with reading comprehension and social manners. Without self esteem, the ability to read and social manners, the youth had very little chance for success in life.

The youth showered, brushed their teeth and dressed in their new attire. Three local barbers patiently waited in the grand room to remove the chaos and confusion of dead cells (hair) from their heads. The youth complained and cursed about getting their hair cut, especially the ones with the dreadlocks, mullets and afros. Getting a haircut for many meant change and change was a very fearful event.

After the barbers shaved and trimmed the last head into a respectable haircut, Hawkinson entered the room. He had just returned from the male staff showers. It was as if he walked into a different facility. The youth looked like well-groomed young men. It was amazing what a haircut, the removal of facial hair and decent clothing did for their appearance and self esteem.

As the barbers walked around with mirrors showing the adolescents their new looks and complimenting them, many of them smiled and stroked the sides of their faces while rubbing the tops of their heads. It was as if a light flickered in their eyes, giving them a sense of hope. Hawkinson believed self-esteem and motivation began with one's appearance. When a person dresses good, they tend to look good, when they look good, they tend to feel good, and when they feel good, they tend to do good.

Hawkinson sat back *hawking* or observing their every move. Studying their characters always gave Hawkinson a head start at growing to know them. A teen with hazel eyes just had his thick, golden dreadlocks cut off. He sat alone frowning. It was as if someone stole his bike, best friend and lunch money all at the same time. By the look on his face, Hawkinson could tell he disliked his new look.

"You okay youth Marley Averson," Hawkinson asked reading the youth's temporary nametag.

"Man, this haircut stuff is for the birds. Y'all might as well call my probation officer and tell her to come get me and take me back to detention, because this is the last time I ever get my haircut," the deviant eyed, somewhat overweight youth said with an upside down smile. The pupils of his eyes turned coal black as he grew angry. It was something Hawkinson had never seen in any of the youth in all the cycles of working at Lake Apache.

"Give it some time to grow on you youth Averson, just give it some time," Hawkinson said as he walked away observing the other youth closely.

Although Hawkinson was an optimist, he knew it was only a matter of time before one apple in the barrel decided to shift the positive moment into a negative one. Sure enough, a Puerto Rican youth from the east coast with soft wavy hair decided to have a little roast before lunch. He zoomed in on Joby Kiddwell's tight course hair and began his roasting session.

"Hey dawg, we just got hair cuts and you still look like you got B.B. King and the million man march on your head. You got all those little knotty soldiers lined up in a row. Nigga your hair is so tight it's screamin' Marvin Gaye's mercy, mercy me." The room went into an uproar. At first Joby seemed to be a good sport about the comment. He rubbed his course hair and nodded his head with a half smile trying his best not to show embarrassment. Pumped up and charged from the laughs he was getting from his peers, the Puerto Rican youth lit into Joby again.

"Damn dawg, these kinky naps are tighter than the joints I used to roll," he said raising his fingers up to his lips and licking them. The room went into an uproar once more. One of the male rookie youth counselors made a move as if he was going to break up the commotion. Hawkinson shook his head and signaled for his comrade not to interfere. The counselor backed down.

Feeling disrespected and humiliated, Joby was no longer smiling. He was looking at the Puerto Rican youth with a hateful eye. The youth continued with his roast. He hurled insult after insult at his peer. Finally when the Puerto Rican youth turned away to laugh it up with another peer, Joby leaped from his seat and shot after him like a rocket.

Inches before Joby reached the youth, another youth named Geronimo jumped up in an attempt to grab Joby, but he was too late. Joby launched a punch barely missing his peer's head. Feeling the air buzzing by the side of his head, the youth quickly stood. Joby fought relentlessly to free himself from the grasp of Geronimo as he cursed the Puerto Rican youth like a sailor. The Puerto Rican youth laughed in an antagonistic manner as he placed his hand on Joby's forehead.

"Calm down little man, you and these little bad ass soldiers," he said rubbing his hand across Joby's course hair while laughing it up. Joby continued to try and free himself. Hawkinson stepped forward with a whistle between his lips and blew into it as loud as his lungs would allow. The sound of the whistle echoed throughout the large room. Everyone stopped what they were doing and focused their attention in his direction. Some of the youth covered their ears from the reverberating noise.

He pointed and motioned for Joby to return to his seat. After youth Geronimo released him, the hostile Joby stormed out of the room kicking and tossing empty chairs from his path. Hawkinson silently pointed to the Puerto Rican youth to have a seat. Sunflower had just returned from the female dormitory. She stood at the entrance with her arms folded observing what was taking place.

With a smirk on his face, the Puerto Rican youth attempted to stare Hawkinson down. Hawkinson looked directly into the eyes of the youth with his bold stare and read his intentions. The youth was no match in a staring contest with the wise, humble disciplinarian. Reading the seriousness in Hawkinson's eyes, the youth took his seat and looked away in a frustrated manner before returning his gaze to Hawkinson.

"Focus up," Hawkinson said to the entire group. "We do not use the term nigga here, ever. Nor do we use any other derogatory terms to belittle the next man to big ourselves up," he said looking through the Puerto Rican youth's eyes directly at his soul. "If you want to use the word for expressing your feelings, use it in your personal journal located on the desk in your room. If that term is used again, we will all be writing a five-page error-free essay on why we choose to use the word, and then we will discuss it in a marathon group. Do I make myself clear?" he asked the group of confused youth. For most of the youth, the "N" word was a part of their everyday vocabulary. However, Hawkinson and his colleagues excluded the word from the place of higher learning. It had no place there. None of the youth had a response. "I said do I make myself clear!" Hawkinson asked again slightly elevating his thunderous voice.

"Yeah," most of the youth said simultaneously.

"We have afternoon meal in exactly ten minutes. If these two youth do not find a way to resolve their issues with or without your help, we will postpone mealtime until the issue is resolved," Hawkinson said looking in the direction of Joby who was standing in the hallway with clinched fists.

"Man that's a bunch of bullshit," one of the other youth mumbled. Some of the youth began smacking their lips and rolling their eyes as they agreed with their peer's comment.

"How many females do we have in here?" Hawkinson asked. The youth looked around the room in confusion. "No females?" he asked stepping into the center of the grand room slightly shimmying. When Hawkinson's passion intensified, the energy inside grew quite animated. He would sometimes shimmy his shoulders and use his hands quite often to express himself. For many of his colleagues it was quite humorous.

"Then I shouldn't hear any lips smacking and see any eyes rolling. As future men, we need not smack our lips and roll our eyes to make a point. If you would like to challenge the comment I made about mealtime, then raise your hand and speak out... like future men."

One brave soul chose to raise his hand high into the air. Hawkinson spotted the youth and motioned for him to speak. The thin youth with deep pigmentation and high cheek bones stood on his feet with his barely visible chest stuck out and jaws tight.

"Why do the rest of us have to suffer for the actions of those two?" he asked pointing at his peers.

"What is your name sir?" Hawkinson asked.

"It sho in the hell ain't sir," the youth replied with an attitude as he gave one of his peers next to him a pound. Some of his peers chuckled at the response while rooting him on. Ten cycles ago as a rookie, Hawkinson would have been all over the youth for making such a response, but times had changed and so had he. He'd grown and matured. The slice of humble pie he had every morning with a tall glass of joy grounded him deeply. Hawkinson was much wiser and tolerant, which made him much more responsive than reactive.

"Then are you a ma'am?" Hawkinson asked as he raised one of his naturally arched eyebrows. Some of the youth cracked up laughing at Hawkinson's response.

"Hell naw I ain't no ma'am," the youth shamefully said as he looked around the room to see which peers were laughing at him.

"Non-verbal!," Sunflower called out to the group. The group silenced themselves, but not before one of the youth named LaBoy looked her up and down and licked his lips. Sunflower noticed him from her peripheral. She chose to let it slide for the moment, but would definitely confront him later. Hawkinson knew a clown couldn't perform if he had no audience. His plan was to quickly step into the spotlight as the ringmaster and shut down the entertainment.

"Then if you're not a sir or a ma'am, what and who are you?" he asked with piercing eyes. The youth paused for a moment and looked away before returning his gaze to the one they called Hawk.

"Lil' No Good is my name and chumping fools up who talk smack is the name of my game," he said with a hint of sarcasm.

"Tell his ass cuz," one of his peers said. Hawkinson remained under the spotlight as he sliced right in with a comeback of his own.

"Well Mr. No Good, I use fools for fuel and bring shame to their pathetic game, now stop chasing the cool and tell me, what is your cute little birth name?" he asked as he approached and stood before the youth. Ooohs and aaahs filled the room.

"Get at him shorty, show him how we get down in DOC," another peer said in the background.

"We can do without the remarks from the children's choir," Sunflower added. The youth whom Hawkinson was challenging tried to think of a comeback. He hadn't expected Hawkinson to match his wits so quickly. He had nothing, so he humbly surrendered.

"Roosevelt... Roosevelt Franklin," he said his name in a low tone. Some of his peers snickered at the name. Hawkinson read the embarrassment in the youth's eyes. He knew he was being honest.

"Okay Mr. Franklin, I thank you for your honesty and regardless of what you have been led to believe, you are not Lil No Good. Take the negative label off yourself. If you think you're no good, then that's exactly what you'll be for the rest of your days on this earth. I called you sir, because the term is one of high respect. When I refer to you all as *Sirs*, I am letting you know how much I respect you. Do you all overstand?" Hawkinson asked scanning the room.

"Yeah," Roosevelt and some of his peers said in low voices, avoiding eye contact as they hung their heads. The persistent disciplinarian asked them again. This time the group responded in a louder tone.

"The answer to youth Roosevelt's question is that we all suffer the consequences of our peers' actions because we are all responsible for one another. If we can all laugh together, then we can all work together to resolve the current issue. Here at Lake Apache Academy you are your brother's keeper. What is your name sir?" Hawkinson asked the Puerto Rican youth. "Birth name?" he asked, quickly reading the youth's thoughts before he spoke. The youth lowered his head.

"Manuel Sanchez," he said softly.

"Speak up sir so that we can hear you," Hawkinson commanded. Manuel repeated his name in a much louder voice.

"We can work together to resolve the issue that youth Manuel and youth Joby created. Violence is unacceptable here. There's plenty of that where you came from. If we must fight, let us fight for a greater cause like keeping you sirs out of the penitentiaries and graveyards. When this issue has been dealt with appropriately, then we will proceed to line up and walk in a single file line over to the dining hall." Without prompt, Manuel stood up and approached Joby with his hand held out. Joby stared at the outstretched hand of his peer for a moment before slapping him five.

"My bad on the hair thing, you cool?" Manuel asked with a slight smirk.

"Yeah," Joby responded without looking at him. Manuel looked over at Hawkinson in a condescending manner as he walked back to his seat. Hawkinson knew the level of sincerity from Manuel was low, but it was okay for the time being. His message to the youth was loud and clear.

Chapter 2

Orientation

(Problem Solving 101)

As the youth walked from the living quarters to the dining hall they observed the female residents and younger male youth from other units walk in single file lines to their destinations. The August sun was beaming down. The temperature was already in the mid nineties.

"Got us out here like we in a chain gang or boot camp," Franklin whispered to Sanchez.

"More like slavery," Sanchez whispered in return.

"Hey homey, they must got me mistaken for fairy Larry or somebody being up in here with all you hard legs. This aint gonna work. I gots to get me one of dem honey dips over there," said a tall thin youth with a strong southern dialect. His name was Brennen and he nearly sprung his neck trying to look at the females. A few of his peers chuckled.

"Man you better chill before ol' Hawkeyes catch you and beam the spotlight on you like he just did Franklin and Sanchez. My cousin who was here three years ago told me that Hawk reads minds like Professor Xavier from the X-men," the youth said.

"Man, ain't nobody scared of ol' beady black eyed peas Hawkeyes," said Brennen. *"I use fools for fuel and bring shame to their pathetic game,"* he said mocking Hawkinson.

"Youth Brennen step out of the line," Hawkinson called out from far back.

"You either stupid or been smokin' crack. Whatever you do, don't look in his eyes," Sanchez told Brennen, as he kept moving.

"Damn, how'd he hear that?" Brennen whispered to himself with a face of terror as he stepped out of line. The other Unit 8 youth passing by gave Brennen a look as if he was headed for the gas chamber.

"You like staring down the honey dips?" Hawkinson asked approaching.

"I-I-I, ugh, I was just."

"You were just what youth Brennen?"

"I was just saying I hope we having honey for lunch to dip our, ugh, you know, our celery sticks in," the youth said refusing eye contact.

"Is that what you eat where you're from youth Brennen?"

"Yes sir, that's what we eat all the time," he said looking up at the sky.

"Where are you from Brennen?" Hawkinson asked.

"Sir, I'm from Kentucky."

"What part of Kentucky?" Hawkinson asked studying the youth's wandering eyes.

"Louisville, sir," he said refusing eye contact.

"Youth Brennen, if I ever hear you refer to dipping anything in honey as long as you're on this campus we're going to have some problems. Are we clear, sir?"

"Clear as Lake Apache," Brennen said gulping as he looked towards the lake in the distance.

"Good, now get in line so you can eat sir. Don't want you to miss out on your celery sticks and honey," Hawkinson said with a raised eyebrow. The youth joined his peers at the end of the line. Sunflower approached Hawkinson.

"Celery sticks and honey, that was pretty creative. I might have to try that," she said smiling. Meanwhile, the group of girls Brennen was staring at were approaching. Hawkinson rested his hands behind his back. "Morning ladies," he said nodding his head at the female youth.

"Good morning," some of the female youth said simultaneously as they looked down at the ground. Others chose not to speak due to their lack of social manners. There were the few that smiled flirtatiously; happy to get the attention of a male.

The male and female youth at Lake Apache could not socialize with each other until the last phase, which was the blue phase. The first two phases were about focusing on their treatment issues. Once they were on the blue phase, they could attend a coed luncheon that took place once a week and was supervised by the senior staff.

*　　*　　*　　*　　*

The Unit 8 youth entered the dining hall and sniffed the air. The smell of burgers, french fries, corn and chocolate chip cookies lingered. Each table had nametags on it and some of the youth began to celebrate by high fiving when they discovered they were sitting with someone they liked. Others who didn't like the assigned seating arrangement sighed and developed attitudes as they mean mugged the staff.

"Ay man, why we gotta sit like this?" one of the youth asked Mr. Minnis. Minnis was a very humorous man, but when approached the wrong way, he could be highly confrontational. He had a reputation across the campus as being a jokester, which many felt was the polar opposite of Hawkinson.

"A is the first letter in the alphabet, B is the second, so before you address me, I "C" you're going to need a lesson in mannerism 101," Minnis said approaching the youth.

"Cuz got nursery rhymes," the youth said to his peers at the table with an antagonistic smile.

"Stand up," Minnis commanded with a smile. The youth looked up at him and dropped his smile. He slowly stood. "What's your name son?"

"B-nizzle," the youth said in a confident cool manner.

"I don't mean your Sesame Street name, your birth name please, sir."

"Oh, you mean my slave name."

"That'll do just as well," Minnis said while still smiling, refusing to feed into the youth's wit.

"Braylon...Braylon Nicholson," the youth said.

"Braylon, when you address me, please address me as Mr. Minnis, not cuz, bruh, homey or anything else. Are we clear on that?"

"Yeah, we're clear Dennis the Minnis...oops my bad... I mean, Mr. Minnis," he said looking over at his peers who were trying not to laugh. "And when you address me, address me as Braylon, because I ain't never yo' son," he said with an air of cockiness.

"I didn't call you son because you're mine, I called you *sun* because you shine brightly. If you don't believe me just ask Mr. Hawkinson, he'll give you a nice little metaphorical lesson on the sun shining and the clouds being gray and all that happy good stuff," Minnis said with a comical smile as he tugged at the lower part of his shirt as he so often did when speaking. "Now sit down Braylon, so you can be called up to get your Lake Academy version of the happy meal. Who knows, the meal might even come with a little anger management toy." The youth hesitated at first. "Go ahead, its okay, Braylon," Minnis said still smiling as he backed away. Braylon flopped down in his seat. Minnis looked around the room to see if anyone else wanted to challenge him.

"Anybody else want to know why we have assigned seats? Speak now or forever hold your peace. I have nothing but time," Minnis said looking at the watch on his wrist.

"Sit yo' lame ass down!" one of the youth shouted across the dining hall.

"Well thanks to the smart guy across the way, I'm going to take a few minutes of your time and tell you why we have seating arrangements." A large number of the youth sighed and focused their attention on the youth across the room. They sensed that Minnis could be long-winded with his speeches.

"Yo' dumb ass started all of this," LaBoy mumbled to Braylon. Braylon stood up to challenge LaBoy.

"Yo' mama is a dumb ass… dumb ass!" he said clutching his fists. LaBoy held his peace, only because he knew it would prolong mealtime. He humbled his tongue until a later time.

"Is there a problem youth Braylon?" Minnis asked.

"This heartless coward called me a dumb ass," he said staring LaBoy down.

"Well are you?" Minnis asked.

"Are you?" Braylon asked with a bitter tone as he focused his misguided anger towards Minnis.

"I guess I would be if I responded to someone calling me a dumb ass, but since I didn't…I guess I'm not," Minnis said with the same humorous grin. Braylon sat and slumped down in his chair.

Minnis went on to explain to the group why seating arrangements were created. He purposely took his time, which added a little peer pressure on Braylon. He knew peer pressure could bust a pipe. It was an effective tool. The entire time he spoke, the majority of the youth stared at Braylon who was now staring at the floor. Even the boys at Braylon's table who previously laughed at his antics were now staring at him coldly.

*　　*　　*　　*　　*

After breakfast, the youth returned to the program for more orientation. Handouts of the rules, expectations and the model for treatment were passed out. The treatment model was based on cognitive behavioral therapy, a psychotherapy that focuses on awareness, judgement, assumptions, beliefs and behaviors. The goal of the treatment is to influence negative emotions that relate to the false appraisal of events. Cognitive Behavioral Therapy treats various kinds of mental and emotional disorders including rapid mood swings and anxiety. While in therapy, each of the youth were issued a journal to record important events, feelings, thoughts, assumptions and beliefs that might be unhelpful or unrealistic. Their journals would become their daily reference guide. Relaxation and meditation techniques were also included in the therapy process.

During the orientation, some stared off into space while others nodded and fought to stay awake. Some drew gang graffiti on the handouts before making paper airplanes out of them. After orientation, Hawkinson announced that there would be a test on the handout at 1400hrs and those who passed were going to the sports complex for basketball and recreation.

The youth who were previously spacing out instantly sat up and focused when they heard basketball. The nodding youth woke up and the youth making paper airplanes straightened out their papers and began reading.

Basketball to most of the young men was like drugs to an addict. They craved it. They had to have it, and would do almost anything to get their hands on the round ball, even take a test they had no interest in taking. They split up into five groups of six during the study period. Most studied diligently while a few goofed around playing the dozens and telling Yo' Momma jokes. Only half the youth would go on to pass the test. The half who passed were taken to the complex as promised. The others stayed back for study hall and more orientation.

Hawkinson and his supporting cast split the youth into two teams for a game of basketball. After laying down the rules, Hawkinson met the two captains in the center of the court for the tip off. Braylon and Brennen were chosen as captains. The first team to reach a score of twelve by ones and two's would hail victor.

Although Braylon was a good five to six inches shorter than his peer, he won the tip. He tipped the ball to a peer, who in return passed the ball back to him. Braylon dribbled the ball up to the three-point line and pulled up for a jumper without bothering to look for his teammates. As a coach, right away Hawkinson observed Braylon's skills along with his selfishness.

"Swish," Braylon said along with the sound of the net as he smiled. It was the first real smile he displayed since arriving to Lake Apache. He back peddled up the court with his teammates and waited for the other team to bring the ball up court. Before the other team could advance the ball beyond half court, Braylon sprinted forward and snatched the ball from the opposing player. He dribbled down with defenders in pursuit. The five foot eight inch Braylon threw the ball off the backboard and caught it with one hand, slamming it in the goal. Just like that, his team was up 3-0.

Braylon acted as if he was heading back down court. When the other team threw the ball in bounds, the speedy youth stole it out of mid air. He avoided the easy lay up and dribbled out to the three-point line putting up another shot that hit nothing but net. Braylon was a one-man show. Sunflower looked at Hawkinson and shook her head.

This went on until his team was up 7-0. LaBoy scolded his peers and demanded they let him guard Braylon. The frustrated youth tried his best to keep up with the savvy basketball player, but the lightning quick Braylon proved to be too much. He ran circles around LaBoy, and scored on him at will. Out of frustration, the angered LaBoy reflected on the comment Braylon made about his mother being a dumb ass while in the dining hall, which infuriated him even more.

As Braylon brought the ball up court for the game winning shot, one of his peers set a pick for him. Braylon dribbled around the pick and went in for the lay up dunk. The angered LaBoy blasted through the pick and ran across the lane, jumped into the air at the same time as Braylon, while connecting a forceful forearm to his throat.

Braylon released the shot and fell hard to the floor hitting the back of his head and holding his throat while gagging for breath. The ball banked off the backboard and scored. Hawkinson blew the whistle for a flagrant foul as everyone gathered around Braylon.

LaBoy bent down and whispered to Braylon, "That's for talking about my dead Momma. I told you I was gonna get your lame ass." He then stepped over him and walked away. Braylon rolled around on the floor coughing and gagging as tears streamed out the corners of his eyes.

"Youth LaBoy, you're done! Go sit down," Sunflower said before blowing her whistle and pointing towards the bleachers. Hawkinson and a few youth kneeled down to tend to Braylon.

"You're okay. You just had the wind knocked out of you. Relax and breathe slowly," Hawkinson said helping Braylon up off the floor. Slowly, the injured youth stood and began to regulate his breathing. As everyone stepped back to give him space, Braylon pushed by everyone and charged LaBoy who was walking towards the bleachers. Stumbling and staggering, the injured youth caught up to his peer and threw a punch at the back of his head. Had it not been for his peers yelling for him to look out, LaBoy would have caught a serious blow, which would have knocked him out.

He turned around just in time to side step the incoming blow. LaBoy raised his hands, but the mighty blow Braylon launched broke through the block and skinned the side of his forehead. The momentum from Braylon's punch carried through and knocked LaBoy off balance. Both youth crashed hard into the wooden bleachers as they commenced to swinging and swearing.

Hawkinson stood back as Sunflower, two of the rookie male staff and two of the complex employees sprinted over to break up the wrestling match. After the youth separated, Hawkinson blew into the whistle with his powerful lungs until he had everyone's undivided attention.

"Everyone, have a seat on the bleachers," he said to the youth as he walked towards the bleachers in a cool manner. The two complex employees were still holding the struggling Braylon as the two other staff held LaBoy. The other youth sat on the bleachers. Hawkinson approached the bleachers as he stared down LaBoy who was huffing and puffing while wiping away the crimson colored saliva that dripped from his lower lip.

"Problem solving 101!" Hawkinson said shifting his gaze from LaBoy to Braylon. "If you have a problem, solve it without the Neanderthal violence! We cannot go through life throwing punches every time we have a problem. This is the first day of your stay and already there have been two cat fights," he said looking over at Manuel and Joby who lowered their heads.

"We will never see the inside of this complex again if we don't come up with another way to solve our problems!" As Hawkinson was speaking, Sunflower had gone to get paper towels for the two youth to clean themselves up. The discussion on problem solving wasn't just heard by the struggling youth, the many employees at the complex stopped what they were doing and listened in as well. Hawkinson was like E.F. Hutton, when he spoke, everyone seemed to listen.

Chapter 3
The Chief Board of Elder
(From Malehood to Manhood)

Many of the youth continued to struggle with problem solving skills. Instead of using their heads to come up with a positive solution to their many petty issues, a great deal of them continued to resort to verbal threats and physical violence, which was a major part of their past environments. The behaviors reminded Hawkinson of the early days of his career at Lake Apache.

A couple of the youth had already earned a trip back to the Department of Corrections due to their extreme physical violence. The clinical team decided to step it up a notch. They cancelled all trips indefinitely to the sporting complex and other campus facilities except for the dining hall and school.

After school the youth returned to the living quarters where they participated in a concentrated treatment plan (CTP). This plan focused primarily on self-esteem, self-worth and self-respect. After a couple of hours of CTP, the youth attended an exercise program consisting of team building outdoor exercises. Afterwards they participated in the Indian run around the track. Those refusing to participate prolonged their restrictions. Those who cooperated completed the plan in five days. Manuel Sanchez, Scotland Brennen, Roosevelt Franklin, Geronimo Coltrane, Marley Averson and two other youth were the first seven to complete CTP. In honor of their achievements, the youth attended a ceremony. They wore their dress clothes and attended a special feast.

Inspired by their peers' actions and the meal they feasted on, most of the other youth earned their way off restriction a few days later. Even though some of the youth refused to get on board the treatment train, Hawkinson could see and feel a change on the unit. Things were starting to take a turn for the better— so it seemed.

*   *   *   *   *

The time had come for the first Chief Board of Elders ceremony of the young cycle. The ceremony was the heart of treatment. All treatment progress, assignments and phases went through the board of elders. Hawkinson and Minnis both sat on the board as chief elders. As the youth progressed in treatment, three of them would replace the chief elders by earning the right to sit on the board before their peers and conduct the ceremony.

The ceremony began with the youth standing and reciting the Unit 8 Warrior's pledge. After the pledge, they sat and focused their attention on the two Chief Elders. Next, the elders acknowledged the youth that earned privileges for that week. They then called up to the podium the youth who were presenting assignments. Afterwards, the youth who earned consequences were addressed. Closing remarks and encouraging words to the youth by the elders ended the ceremony.

*   *   *   *   *

It was Sunday afternoon in the middle of fall. The skies were blue and the sun was warm and bright. The leaves in the trees had already changed from green to shades of orange, red and yellow. Hawkinson drove with his sunroof open. The leaves fell from the trees and drifted all about. The scene was heavenly beautiful. Hawkinson had thoughts of driving until sunset, even with the price of gas climbing towards the five dollars a gallon mark.

He pulled into the parking lot listening to a track by Brothers Johnson entitled *Strawberry Letter 22*. The song complimented the bright scenery of a grove of trees that stretched across the academy's lawn. Sunflower was standing in the parking lot unloading bags from her car. The sun beamed down on her bronze Arizona complexion, which illuminated her aura.

Hawkinson pulled up next to her playing the music. She smiled and shook her head. He parked the car and shut off the engine, while allowing one of the best songs of all times to continuously flow through the sunroof.

"Is that your theme music Hawk?" Sunflower asked after the song ended.

"Sure is. Everyone should have theme music, even you," he said exiting and locking his car.

"Okay, if I had a theme song Hawk, what would it be?"

"It'd be the theme song to speed racer. I've seen the way you drive," he said taking a couple of bags from her to carry.

"Whatever Hawk. There's nothing wrong with my driving."

"Danica Patrick doesn't take corners the way you do. She's like Morgan Freeman in Driving Miss Daisy compared to you."

*   *   *   *   *

Later that late afternoon Hawkinson and a rookie colleague supervised a group of youth as they raked and bagged fallen leaves out in the grove. A portable stereo player sitting nearby on a picnic table played the song, *I Got Work to Do*, by Ronnie Isley and the Isley brothers. Hawkinson had radioed Sunflower to bring more supplies. The free spirited Maya Sunflower strolled across the freshly cut lawn carrying garbage bags and rakes.

"It's nice to see things are finally coming together out here Hawk," she said approaching and handing the youth the materials.

"Have to give credit to the hard working youth," Hawkinson said closely observing the youth as he always did.

"I have to admit, they've made a tremendous turnaround since the brawl at the complex," she said smiling as she turned and walked away.

Sunflowers are solar flowers that have a strong connection to the sun. The sunflower turns to face the sun as the glowing orb makes its way across the sky. The nature of the subject seemed to reverse when it came to Maya. The sun appeared to follow her and illuminate the essence of her aura as she walked along the path of autumn leaves.

*   *   *   *   *

It was later on during the week. Hawkinson facilitated a group. The topic of discussion was "Malehood to Manhood". He sat at the head of the horseshoe shaped group of youth. He sat back and allowed the youth to develop rules and guidelines to structure the group process. His philosophy was when the youth structured the group with their own rules, they were more apt to follow the rules and respect the group process.

After the rules were in place, the youth voted amongst one another for group leaders. The process began smoothly. Within a matter of minutes, it grew chaotic and unstructured as egos flew. Hawkinson allowed the chaos to play out as he and the group co-facilitator, Mr. Minnis sat back and observed. Finally, youth Braylon stood up and whistled. Everyone stopped talking. He began pointing and assigning his peers to different tasks. When he finished, only LaBoy stood and challenged his decisions.

"Dude, who died and made you boss?" the hefty LaBoy asked.

"Apparently not you doughboy," Braylon said with a sarcastic smirk.

"Why do you always think you're better than everybody?" youth LaBoy asked Braylon.

"Not everybody, just you…doughboy," he said with the same smirk.

"I got your doughboy, right here," LaBoy said grabbing the crotch of his pants as he stood and began making his way towards Braylon. Geronimo and Brennen stood up to put a halt to LaBoy's forward progress by putting a hand on his chest.

"Dude I will whup yo punk ass," youth LaBoy said as he tried to push his way through youth Geronimo while pointing at Braylon in a violent manner. Hawkinson and Minnis continued to observe. Problem solving 101 was the theme of the program and they were allowing the youth to solve their problems. The other youth in the group sat back and observed. Some appeared intimidated by the sudden shift in energy, while a few others chuckled to cover up their own anxiety and fear.

"Stop it! Look at you two! No wonder we can't go to the complex or do anything else! We can't even organize simple little rules for a group without the two of you acting like a couple of children," Geronimo said in his proper frustrated tone. "All you do is argue and fight! The bullshit stops now," he said looking from one peer to the next. The room grew silent. No one uttered a word. Hawkinson smiled internally.

"Sit down and let's do this the right way," youth Geronimo told his two arguing peers. Both youth looked at Geronimo in disbelief. "I'm not playing, I said sit down," he said elevating his voice. Both youth slowly backed off and sat down. Hawkinson and Minnis were both amazed as they looked at one another and smiled. Hawkinson could feel himself developing goose bumps. He'd been waiting patiently and humbly for that very moment, that moment for one warrior to step up and take charge. Geronimo Coltrane stepped up and grabbed leadership by the horns, and rode it for what it was worth.

Geronimo took over and governed the group with authority. He commanded his peers to write down who they thought would make the best group leaders. It was as if he borrowed a page right out of Hawkinson's book. The motivated youth was slowly learning the definition of leadership in a positive peer culture.

*　　*　　*　　*　　*

After the tallying of the votes, Geronimo and Brennen hailed as victors. Unanimously, their peers voted the two of them as group leaders. Hawkinson was extremely proud of Geronimo's leadership. The rest of his peers were finally starting to get the concept of positive peer culture, at least so it seemed.

Hawkinson and Minnis tag teamed as they discussed the differences between males and men. Hawkinson grew energetically animated as always when his passion began to flow. Most of the youth were under the false impression that a male and a man were one and the same, but they were wrong. Males range in many different age groups. Males have certain physical features and attributes of a man, such as levels of testosterone and that dangling organ between their legs that they think is the guiding golden compass to all their problems. The difference between a male and a man totally depends upon his degree of thinking, the responsibilities he takes on, the courage he displays and the care, concern and respect he displays for others. A man also uses the head between his shoulders to guide him when making crucial decisions and not the one attached to his lower anatomy.

During the group, Hawkinson listened to the youth discuss the false impressions given by others that led them to believe they were men. Selling drugs while carrying around wads of cash was one of the impressions that led them to believe they were men. Having premature sexual intercourse, impregnating females, and not being there for the child was another false impression. Fighting gang wars in the streets and firing bullets in the direction of innocent victims with no care and concern was another false impression. The list went on and on. The youth at Lake Apache Academy were starting to realize the differences between a male and a man. It wasn't the responsibility of Lake Apache's staff to change the youth, it was the adolescents' responsibility to make changes if they wanted to break their vicious cycles.

*   *   *   *   *

As time progressed, Hawkinson and his team of colleagues continued to facilitate groups that benefited the youth. Everyday it was starting to look and feel more like a positive peer culture. Even though the petty arguments and fights still occurred, it was nowhere close to what it was like during the first few weeks of the yellow phase. The majority of the youth were starting to adapt to their new environment.

Sunflower and Hawkinson facilitated a group on personal hygiene. The topic of hygiene and discussing male body parts made many of the youth nervous and uncomfortable due to a woman co-facilitating the group. It was as if they morphed into gremlins after eating beyond midnight. They would all but lose their mind. Hawkinson would have to facilitate a pre-group just to get the young men to focus. For some it worked, but for others, no matter what Hawkinson did to prepare them, they just couldn't handle themselves.

During the course of the hygiene group, Hawkinson brought in a male mannequin with anatomically correct body parts and a video. After the video, he and Sunflower randomly selected youth to display the correct way to wash the body and take care of oral hygiene on the mannequin. Of course that was a window of opportunity for some to be highly inappropriate, like youth LaBoy. He was the first to test the waters. He sat up on the edge of his seat with a big wolfish grin.

"Excuse me Ms. Sunflower, but what if one happens to be well endowed or a lot bigger than the average male, how would he go about washing his... you know," he said with a smirk on his face as his eyes dropped below to his genitals. A few of his immature peers chuckled while the more mature ones sighed, shook their heads in disgust and waved him off. Hawkinson shook his head. He felt sorry for youth LaBoy. The troubled teen had no idea what he'd just gotten himself into.

"After you step out of your imagination you can start with some warm water and lots of soap youth LaBoy," she responded with a straight face. The room went into an uproar. It took everything within Hawkinson to keep a straight face. Youth LaBoy eased back in his chair in a real slow manner as he stroked the invisible hairs under his chin. It was obvious that he was embarrassed beyond embarrassment.

"Hey LaBoy, you dropped something," Braylon said pointing to the floor. LaBoy shifted his eyes down to the floor.

"What?" he asked.

"Your face," Braylon said laughing it up. The room went into an uproar once more. Minnis with his humor and comical ways didn't make matters any better as he walked towards youth LaBoy.

"I have some superglue if you want to put that thing back together," he said in a humorous tone of voice. He then pretended to pick pieces of LaBoy's shattered face off the floor and hand it to him. Minnis always had a way of turning a potentially destructive situation into a humorous lighthearted one. LaBoy used Minnis' humor to escape what he was truly feeling. He smiled as he pretended to accept pieces of his face from the smiling Minnis.

After the laughter subsided, the group continued. If there were any youth who had plans of testing Sunflower, those plans went out the window. Her response to youth LaBoy cancelled all reservations. If there was one thing males didn't like, it was having their ego deflated in the public eye of others, especially by a woman. It was at that moment the male youth at Lake Apache Academy earned monumental respect for Ms. Maya Sunflower.

Chapter 4
A Code of Honor

The hygiene group continued as Hawkinson discussed enuresis (bed wetting). Some of the youth were wetting the bed and hiding the sheets in the closets and couldn't understand why their rooms smelled like a porta potty in sweltering heat. It was as if some one was purposely urinating in the vents and ducts.

*　　*　　*　　*　　*

Late one evening after the youth had all gone to bed, Hawkinson sat in his office filling out reports. He listened to a track by Earth, Wind and Fire entitled *Devotion*. There was a soft knock at the door. When he looked up, youth LaBoy was standing in the doorway. His face showed a look of concern.

"Youth LaBoy, what are you doing out of bed sir?"

"The third shift supervisor gave me permission to come talk to you."

"Can it wait 'til morning? I'm trying to get out of here so I can go rest my eyes," Hawkinson said looking at the clock on the wall.

"No sir, not this. It's important." Hawkinson read the sincerity in LaBoy's eyes.

"Come in and have a seat," he said shutting down the computer. LaBoy hesitated before stepping across the threshold into the office. A look of terror appeared on his face. Hawkinson looked up and noticed the youth still standing at the doorway. "Are you going to stand there and hold up the door or are you going to come in and have a seat? I don't have all night son."

"I know you don't sir… it's just that my peers said they'd rather face the boogeyman himself before coming into your office," LaBoy said easing his way into the office across the highly polished floor as if he was walking on eggshells.

"The boogeyman huh, the last I heard it was Mufasa from the Lion King or Professor Xavier from the X-men," he said with a humorous smile.

"Nope, it's still the boogeyman," LaBoy said with a straight face as he crept across the floor.

"That was humor as in like a joke," Hawkinson said shaking his head.

"I didn't laugh because I ain't never known you to joke sir," LaBoy said looking up at the mask of a Mayan headed warrior painted in shades of blue hanging on the wall behind and above Hawkinson's head. Hawkinson followed the youth's eyes to the mask.

"That's my game face," he said facing LaBoy, who was still standing. He invited the youth to take a seat as he put on his focus face. LaBoy eased his way down into the chair. Hawk sat observing the youth for a moment before speaking. LaBoy's eyes darted back and forth all over the office. The nervous youth eye-spied a number of Hawkinson's most prized possessions in a matter of seconds.

"What do you think?"

"About what?" LaBoy asked.

"About the things in this office that you're studying," he said removing the lid from a jar and offering the youth a mint.

"They're nice," he said leaning forward to accept a mint.

"Let me guess. You were either a runner or a look out for the neighborhood hustler."

"How'd you know," LaBoy asked with a surprised look.

"I've seen eyes like yours walk through that door several times in the past. You eyed everything in this office in a matter of seconds before you reached my desk. Without looking, what's on the top shelf on the book shelf over to your right?" Hawkinson asked.

"A bunch of CBT treatment books."

"What color are the feathers on the Native American chief's headdress sitting in the corner behind you?"

"Sandy brown, rusty red and sky blue," LaBoy said without looking over his shoulder.

"Who's standing in the center of that large portrait holding a basketball surrounded by children hanging on the wall to your left?"

"That would be the all star pro-basketball player that led Chicago to six world championships. He was here?" LaBoy asked looking over at the portrait.

"Very impressive, but what's so important that you're keeping me here after hours?" Youth LaBoy looked at Hawkinson with a look of sincerity. It took him awhile, but he eventually expressed what had been eating away at him. Hawkinson leaned up and sat on the edge of his seat. He asked youth LaBoy to repeat what he expressed. The youth repeated his statement.

Hawkinson leaned back in his chair and sighed deeply. What LaBoy disclosed to him was vile and disturbing information, but the counselor had to investigate as he had done many times in the past. The shock of hearing such information wore off cycles ago. The most difficult part was prompting the youth to be open and honest in a group.

Hawkinson walked youth LaBoy back to his dorm room. He went to the third shift supervisor and explained what was taking place. He respectfully asked the supervisor and third shift staff to awaken and gather all the youth and meet him in the grand room. Three out of four of the staff complied. The one staff member who didn't comply was the one Hawkinson observed closely. A few of the youth whom were already sleeping appeared irritated after waking to attend a group at 2200 hours.

"What's going on Mr. Hawkinson? Why are we going to group?" youth Geronimo asked.

"I'll explain as soon as everyone is here," Hawkinson responded as he continued to observe the uncooperative staff. Geronimo and Brennen did a good job corralling their peers. Once all the youth were in the group sitting, Hawkinson asked the third shift to monitor the youth, while he and the supervisor of that shift conducted a room search.

They searched the rooms thoroughly. As Hawkinson searched the rooms, the third shift staff who appeared fidgety and worried watched him instead of the youth. As time ticked away a few of the youth grew agitated.

Hawkinson and the supervisor returned to the grand room. Hawkinson was carrying a navy blue laundry bag that he found stuffed behind a dryer in the laundry room. The youth knew it had to be something serious going on, because Hawkinson never intervened or engaged the youth on third shift, even when he stayed late to finish paperwork.

"Anyone care to tell me what's in this bag?" he asked holding the bag up over his head. No one said a word. A few of the youth began to shift uncomfortably in their chairs. Hawkinson zeroed in on the dead giveaways. He looked at their eyes one by one. The youth lowered their heads and stared at the floor.

"What's the matter, cat got your tongues?" he asked the group. Still, no one said a word. This went on for a while. If there was anything Hawkinson learned from his experience as a counselor, it was that the youth owned a code of honor. No one talked. No one ratted. Not ratting on their peers was an honor code the youth learned from the streets and corrections. Honoring that code is how many of them survived in their past environments.

Hawkinson had a code of his own. His code was the ability to read personality traits by using the Five Factor Model: Openness, Conscientiousness, Extraversion, Agreeableness and Neuroticism, which made up the acronym OCEAN. The openness trait consists of active imagination, art, music, poetry and attentiveness to inner feelings. Conscientiousness consists of carefulness, self-discipline, thoughtfulness and organization. Extraversion consists of assertive, excited, energetic and talkative characters. Agreeable consists of cooperation, social harmony, kindness, sympathy and trust. Neuroticism consists of anger, anxiety, clinical depression, guilt and moodiness.

Hawkinson used the OCEAN model for the past several cycles and it never failed him. Every youth he'd come face to face with fit under the umbrella of one of the personalities. He studied the youths' movements and eyes as he had been doing since that late August. Youth Roosevelt Franklin raised his hand. Hawkinson called upon him.

"Excuse me Mr. Hawkinson, most of us think you're a really cool dude and all and I don't mean any disrespect when I say this, but ain't nobody about to tell you what's in that bag, even if they know. That's just the way it is."

"You're right youth Roosevelt that is the way it is. It's called the code of honor. That code has been around before you and I were born. This is not the Department of Corrections and I am not a correctional officer. This is not the county jail and I am not a deputy sheriff. This is not the streets and I am not a street hustler. This is a treatment center for youth offenders. It is a place of healing, and the role I play is that of a healing practitioner. I am not your enemy or homey. I am your guide. I am your personal treatment gladiator, innovator and motivator cheering you on to success. If you don't buy into treatment then I cannot help you succeed." The room was extremely quiet. Hawkinson asked the youth as he always did, what was the worst thing that could happen to any of them on any given day during their stay at the academy.

"One of us could die," youth Geronimo said speaking out.

"That's right. One or more of you could die," Hawkinson said acknowledging Geronimo. "My goal is to not let any of you die, especially on my watch," he said reaching into the laundry bag and pulling out a shank.

The youth clamored at the sight of the sharp metal object. Hawkinson reached into the bag and retrieved a set of keys to one of the Lake Apache vehicles, a wad of cash held together by a gold money clip and three black sweatsuits. The majority of the youth leaned back in their seats with a look of astonishment as the commotion continued. A few lowered their heads at the sight of the weapon.

"*Bingo*," Hawkinson thought as he watched the youths' heads drop from guilt. It was three youth with neurotic personality traits. The same three that were told by their parole officer that they would return to the Department of Corrections if they had one more verbal or physical outburst. The youth grew extremely uncomfortable as they began shifting in their seats. Two of the three youth shifted their gaze to the third shift staff. The staff had grown extremely uncomfortable. Hawkinson had him labeled as an agreeable personality trait, which made him an easy target for exploitation. Hawkinson already knew how the story was going to unfold.

One of the three youth acting extremely uncomfortable was Braylon Nicholson. Braylon was one of the most talented youth to ever attend Lake Apache Academy. He was also one of the most stubborn.

"Anyone care to share who brought this into our house?" Hawkinson asked as he looked from Braylon to the other two youth and then to the third shift staff who was perspiring and swaying nervously from side to side.

The tightened muscles in Braylon's jaws moved up and down as he sat up on the edge of his chair. His darting eyes moved all around the room searching for a way out. The other two youth appeared nervous and fearful ready to choke and spill their guts at any time.

"Don't you all speak at once," Hawkinson said to the group as he studied the intensifying tension on Braylon's face. The silence was starting to get to a great deal of the youth. Some began fanning their legs nervously. Some chewed away at their fingernails while the more emotionally unstable youth rocked back and forth. Hawkinson knew it was just a matter of time before one of the youth blew like a volcano.

"Do you have something you'd like to share youth Parker?" Hawkinson asked the adolescent who kept looking at the third shift staff. The youth looked up at Hawkinson with wide eyes that were starting to turn red and watery. His bottom lip quivered. Braylon looked over and tried to get Parker's attention, but the youth refused to look his way.

Just as Parker was about to speak, Braylon spoke up and interrupted. He began telling Hawkinson and the entire group how he set up the run attempt. He gave them detail by detail how it would go down. He confessed that he paid the third shift staff the money he earned from working in dietary while locked up in corrections to bring in the shank and the sweat suits.

After Braylon gave the statement, the third shift supervisor called the police. When they arrived, the officers stood back observing the group. Many of the youth became angry and anxious at the sight of the officers, especially the youth who had past issues with the law.

After Braylon was asked to tell his story again, the staff member lowered his head in shame as one of the officers approached him. The officer ordered the staff to place his hands behind his back. Without a struggle, he quietly placed his hands behind his back as the cuffs locked around his wrists. The officer guided him away to one of the nearby offices to read him his rights.

When questioned about whom the extra two black sweatsuits were for, Braylon admitted to asking a couple of his peers to go with him, but as the time grew near for the run attempt to take place, he told the group that the both of them backed out.

"Who were the two youth?" Hawkinson asked as he studied Braylon's eyes.

"Youth Parker and youth Hill," Braylon said looking Hawkinson directly in the eye. Parker and Hill both lowered their heads. Hawkinson knew it was more of a relief on their behalf. He also knew Braylon had just taken the fall for his two peers. Hawkinson had witnessed the game Braylon was playing in past cycles. Observation and experience were his greatest teachers.

Hawkinson asked the two youth if Braylon's story was true. Both youth slowly raised their heads and looked over at Braylon who was staring right through them. He had just protected them with the code of honor. He took the rap for them and for that, he knew someday they both would return the favor at a later time and place.

Both youth agreed before lowering their heads. It was obvious Braylon was chief royalty according to his peers. It was more than just Parker and Hill that revered the youth. It was all of his peers, except for LaBoy. In their eyes, Braylon was their unspoken leader. He always spoke up and took up for them. Braylon presented no fear of anything or anyone. His smooth street talk and knowledge of the system is how he survived. Parker and Hill faced returning to corrections due to lewd behaviors. Braylon set up a run plan. The plan was to return to the harsh street life, which took the place of his mother and father. The streets were the parents that raised him.

Chapter 5
The Snitch

Braylon was sixteen and on probation. Parker and Hill were both eighteen and on parole. It was easy for Braylon to make the sacrifice. He had less to lose due to his legal status and age. Facing new charges as adults for having a weapon, Parker and Hill would both face time in an adult corrections facility.

Braylon studied LaBoy's body language. Judging by his actions, he knew it was his rival who snitched him out. Braylon could feel his blood start to boil under his flesh as he thought back to when LaBoy walked past his room to go to Hawkinson's office. As Hawkinson continued to grill Braylon about his plans to run, the infuriated youth answered each question truthfully and respectfully as possible, as he stared at LaBoy. Underneath his calm demeanor was a flow of hot lava ready to erupt.

All the supervisors and seniors including Minnis and Sunflower received a phone call about the severity of the group, and were asked to report to the campus immediately. When they walked into the grand room, a police officer was leading the arrested third shift staff out of one of the offices in handcuffs to the squad car. Sunflower looked at the staff in disappointment as he lowered his head from guilt.

Even though Braylon admitted to operating on his own will, all the youth had to undergo an interviewing process. It was part of policy and procedure. That's where Minnis shined like a star. He and other supervisors began the process.

Sunflower joined the group and sat in an empty chair near Braylon. He refused to look at her. Along with Hawkinson, she was one of Braylon's biggest advocates in his early stay at Lake Apache. The youth had grown quite fond of both of them. The look on her face showed that she was greatly disappointed in the choices he made.

As Sunflower spoke to the group of young men in a disappointed tone, Hawkinson went into his memory museum where his past thoughts came to life, jumped off the walls and played about. He thought back to the many foolish acts the youth from the past committed at Lake Apache.

Some cycles ago, five youth escaped by stealing a Lake Apache vehicle and ditching it on the south side of Chicago. The vehicle was located, but the youth were not. Months later four out of five of the youth earned a trip to an adult penitentiary for committing another crime. Shortly after that incident, another youth stole a set of keys and lifted a Lake Apache vehicle. The inexperienced youth rolled the vehicle several times in a nearby cornfield. He too served time for felony charges. Another youth escaped out of a bathroom window and ran on foot. He made it to Interstate 57 where he attempted to flag down passing motorists. When he spotted the pursuing staff from Lake Apache, he grew extremely desperate to escape. He jumped onto the hood of a slowing vehicle and began pounding on the windshield screaming that the staff were trying to harm him. The police arrested and detained the youth.

Another set of youth stole bikes from Lake Apache and made it to a nearby mall. Once they arrived, they attempted to hitch a ride from a trucker. The youth concocted a story to the trucker about the physical abuse they suffered from the staff, and needed a ride as far away from the area as possible. Just as the trucker was about to drive the youth away, a local sheriff arrived with a warrant and returned the youth to Lake Apache.

As Hawkinson continued to take a stroll through his active and colorful memory museum, he thought back to a youth who ran frequently from the academy to a nearby town to get his alcohol and drug fix. After the youth would get all boozed up and paint the town red along with his hair, he would return to the academy with a police escort. No matter how many times the youth ran, he always got caught. If not sooner, it was always later.

After Hawkinson exited and locked the door to his memory museum, he scanned the room of the present day youth. Sunflower had just finished addressing the group about her concerns. The tension was starting to build for many. It showed on their faces how worried they were about the future of their leader, Braylon Nicholson and his stay at Lake Apache. Braylon's probation officer faxed a warrant for his arrest. A police officer was standing by to escort him to the Joliet correctional facility for juveniles.

"Youth Braylon, do you have anything to say to your peers before you part ways with them?" Sunflower asked. Still too ashamed to face her, he stood up and stretched as he faced his peers.

"I messed up. Someone could have seriously gotten hurt, or… died as Mr. Hawkinson always says. It's too late to apologize, so verbally I won't, but just know that I do."

The entire body of youth sat silently plugged into Braylon's speech. Even LaBoy who butted heads with him since day one chose to listen. Braylon had a very charismatic way of expressing the thoughts that danced around in his busy mind.

"So before I go, I'd just like to say I did learn something in my short stay here and I do have one goal in mind," he said to his peers. Hawkinson, Sunflower, Minnis, the other staff and youth were all pretty much thinking in the same realm of thought. They thought that Braylon learned a lesson from the act that he committed and his goal would be to someday return to Lake Apache Academy and make things right by finishing the treatment program. They all looked on and listened with anticipation as they waited for Braylon to announce what he learned along with his goal.

"I learned to never trust a snitch and my goal at this moment is to knock LaBoy the f--- out," he said turning towards LaBoy with swiftness and throwing a series of Mississippi haymakers. As soon as Braylon's closed fist made contact with LaBoy's open face, the crimson river of life flowed from his lips, nose and upper eye. Due to the calmness of his speech, no one expected his response. Everyone was in shock. This was a typical Braylon Nicholson move. He knew all along what he was going to do and that is why he couldn't look Sunflower in the eyes during the group.

Spattered in LaBoy's red river of life and still too shocked to move were the youth sitting next to him. Braylon's fist moved super fast as if he'd temporarily stepped outside of the matrix of existence. LaBoy attempted to cover his face with his arms to keep the incredibly heavy blows from causing more damage. The force of Braylon's punches broke through LaBoy's arms and continued to connect with LaBoy's face. Swear words rolled off Braylon's tongue each time he threw a punch. The words slapped LaBoy violently in his ears.

After the momentary shock wore off, Minnis, Sunflower, Hawkinson and a couple of other staff jumped in and pulled Braylon off LaBoy, but by that time the damage was complete. LaBoy's lips, nose and eyes instantly began to swell. His nose looked like a red bell pepper. His eyes and lips looked as if he had been in a fight with Rocky I, II, III and IV all at the same time.

"You're a trick snitch!" Braylon shouted at LaBoy as he continuously tried to get at him. A third shift staff directed the many confused and startled youth out of the grand ballroom into another area. After staff removed Braylon out of the sight of LaBoy, he immediately stopped fighting. It was as if someone shut off his on switch. His mission was complete.

He calmly placed his hands behind his back and turned his back towards the waiting officer, silently giving him the okay to cuff him. He looked Sunflower in the eyes for the first time that evening. She looked at him in return. For a brief moment, she read the sincere apology in his warm spirit beyond the cold emotionless gaze in his eyes. Braylon then shifted his eyes toward Hawkinson who was standing nearby. The humble Hawkinson approached Braylon slowly and placed his hands on his shoulders to look him square in the eye.

"Volition, we are responsible for the choices we make. This is what you chose, is it not?" he asked. Youth Braylon lowered his head and nodded. "Are you prepared to accept the consequences of your actions?" Once again, the youth nodded yes. "If placed in the same or a similar situation, would you have made the same choice?" Hawkinson asked. Braylon looked up at him with the same distant emotionless gaze. He paused before nodding his head yes.

"I respect your honesty youth Braylon. Have no regrets about the choices you have made. Live with them and let them be learning experiences for your future. When you are ready…if you are ever ready… we'll be here," he said touching the fiery side of the angry youth's face with the coolness of his hand.

The youth instantly tensed up. Hawkinson could tell that he wasn't accustomed to appropriate touch. Silently in his thoughts, Braylon wanted Hawkinson to keep his hand glued to his face. It felt natural in the most appropriate, supportive way. It was as if the magical touch from Hawkinson's aura was healing him upon contact. The disgruntled youth fought hard to hold back the tears he hadn't released since he was five years old.

Sunflower looked away to keep from growing emotional. Hawkinson removed his hand from the youth's face and took a step back. Braylon's head automatically lingered towards the direction of Hawkinson's hand as if it was a magnet.

"Okay son, it's time to go," the officer said. With eyes as dry as the Sahara desert, Braylon lowered his head.

"After all these years Hawk, I don't know how you still do it. Me and the boys down at the station have the greatest respect for you. There's no way in hell I could ever do your job," the officer said. Hawkinson shook the officer's hand and thanked him for the compliment before he guided Braylon away.

LaBoy stood slowly and stumbled around nearly slipping in his own blood that covered an area of the tile floor of the grand room. His revenge was to see Braylon escorted out in cuffs. A couple of staff wearing safety gloves immediately sat him back down before attending to his wounds.

The blood on the floor made the situation appear a lot worse than what it actually was.

When Braylon and the officer stepped outdoors, the sky was pouring down rain. No longer able to hold back his tears, the emotionally challenged youth opened the floodgates. There was no one around to witness his pain, except for the elements of nature. His sizzling tears of anger blended in with the cool raindrops. Braylon looked up at the dark heavens as if he was looking for an answer.

Thoughts of what if and regrets darted in and out of the blackness of his mind. He was torn. A part of him wanted to stay at Lake Apache and test the waters of this thing called treatment. The other part of him wanted to return to his habitat, the concrete jungle. The concrete jungle is where his animalistic nature kicked in. He lived like a beast inside the jungle, free to roam and partake in beastly behaviors.

The officer opened the back door of the squad car and guided Braylon in by the back of his head. The scene was all too familiar to the youth. He had lost count of how many times he'd been arrested. As the officer closed the back door, Braylon focused his attention to the unit eight building.

The remorseful, teary eyed youth used his forehead to clear the steam from the window. Inside one of the windows of the building, he could see the silhouettes of his peers looking out at him. Realizing what he was leaving behind, the tears began to flow heavily from his ducts. For the first time in his life he actually felt like he was part of a special brotherhood.

The officer ignited the engine of the squad car. He then called into the dispatcher and informed her that he was driving to Joliet for a drop off at the youth correctional facility. Braylon continued to watch his peers in the window as the car pulled away and disappeared out of sight.

*   *   *   *   *

Several days later as things returned to normal, the youth on unit eight distanced themselves from LaBoy. No one wanted to associate with a backstabbing snitch. Whenever his name came up, his peers would all refer to him as the snitch. The labeling had gotten so out of control, Hawkinson had to call a group to address the issue.

After the group, Geronimo and Brennen slowly began to integrate LaBoy back into the milieu, but the other youth kept him at a distance. They did not trust him one bit. Some of the staff members including Sunflower chose to speak up in LaBoy's defense about safety on the program.

*   *   *   *   *

One evening during a cooking group held by Sunflower for a small group of the youth, LaBoy displayed why it was so difficult for his peers to engage in relationship building with him. While Sunflower had her back to them pre-warming the oven, LaBoy was sizing her up. He tapped one of his peers on the arm and pointed at Sunflower before licking his lips. The other peer smiled and gave LaBoy a pound. Joby gritted his teeth and shot LaBoy a scowl.

When Sunflower turned around to instruct the youth, she noticed the lustful look in LaBoy's eyes. She also noticed the scowl Joby displayed towards LaBoy. She continued to instruct the class, but raised her awareness and kept her back away from LaBoy. Sunflower was ahead of the game. There had been several youth in the past who attempted to objectify her lustfully as LaBoy had. When the time was right, she would check him as she did before.

After the food was prepared, the youth sat around the table with Sunflower enjoying the meal. LaBoy made comment after comment to Sunflower about how good the meal was as he licked his fingers and sucked on his bottom lip. As he sat across from her, he allowed his foot to ease over to her side underneath the table in attempts to play footsy.

When Sunflower felt his foot touch hers, she immediately asked him to move his foot and leave the table. LaBoy chuckled as he slid his foot back over to his side. Joby was growing impatient with LaBoy's antics.

"Dude, why don't you stop being inappropriate and just leave the table like Ms. Sunflower told you to," Joby said eyeing LaBoy.

"Why don't you go back to eating your baby carrots, and stay out of grown folks business. Shouldn't you be over there at the little kids table anyway holdover," LaBoy shot back with an antagonistic grin. Joby flinched as if he was about to hit LaBoy. Sunflower grabbed him by the wrist.

"Hey, that's enough. Both of you stop right now," she said coaxing Joby down. "Youth LaBoy, put your plate away and leave the table," Sunflower said as she continued to hold Joby's wrist.

"Put my plate away and leave the table. Don't be talking to me like I'm one of these little ass kids."

"Dude, that's a lady you're talking to. You need to watch your mouth," Geronimo said from across the table.

"You watch it for me," LaBoy said dropping his fork in the middle of his plate and sliding the plate aside in a cool manner as if he was giving Geronimo an invitation. The youth sitting next to LaBoy rested his hand on his shoulder to calm him down. LaBoy smacked the youth's hand away.

"So what does that make you a tough Tony or Billy Bad Ass, because you dropped your fork in the middle of your plate?" Geronimo asked.

"Why don't you come over here and find out how tough I am," LaBoy said as he stood. Geronimo, the martial artist, stood only to defend himself as he smiled the entire time.

"No thank you La*Boy*, I saw how tough you were about a week ago when Braylon put the hammers on you," he said adding emphasis to the boy in his name. "I have much better things to do…like the dishes. If another person has the power to make me angry, that means he controls me," he said smiling as he began clearing the table. Geronimo knew he could have fed into LaBoy's boyish games and defeated him easily, but he learned from Hawkinson that the one who remained in control of his emotions always won the battle. The comment infuriated LaBoy.

"There you go copying Mr. Hawkinson. He's always feeding y'all that bullshit and your dumb ass is always eating it up. Hawk ain't nobody. Just like all you lames," LaBoy said pointing closely to Geronimo and Joby's face trying to provoke them.

"It would behoove you to remove your hand from my face," Geronimo said in a calm tone as he continued to smile. Sunflower removed the radio from her hip and called one of the male staff into the kitchenette area.

"See, there you go again sounding like Hawk. Hawk got all you punk ass tricks brainwashed with that calm, cool and collective bullshit. That shit don't work on a beast like me. What kind of name is Geronimo for a black ass house Negro like you anyway? On growth and development and everything I love, I ought to whup yo Ritchie Rich suburbanite talking ass right now," he said stepping towards Geronimo. Before Sunflower could step in between LaBoy and Geronimo, Joby picked up a plate and smashed it over LaBoy's head.

"I'm tired of you starting shit! You always starting shit!" Joby was like a short fused firecracker. He was yelling and screaming like an untamed animal as he went after LaBoy. Two male staff stepped into the kitchenette area. One of them the size of a defensive lineman grabbed Joby in a basket hold from behind and attempted to pull him out of the situation. The thin but strong youth began kicking and swinging wildly. He kicked the table as dishes and food flew in several different directions. Several youth from a nearby room came running to the scene when they heard Joby yelling and screaming.

Learning that LaBoy was once again the source of the chaos, the other youth wanted to jump him as well. The youth were still angry with LaBoy for the absence of Braylon, which was the real reason for wanting to fight him. The other male staff attempted to block the angry youth from getting into the kitchenette and tearing LaBoy apart.

Several of the youth were swearing while repeatedly yelling snitch as they attempted to push past the counselors. LaBoy began yelling at the top of his lungs and reciting gang terminology. He flashed multiple gang signs at his peers who were trying to get into the room. A staff member called code blue. Soon, staff from other programs rushed to the scene for support. It took a while for the mini riot to be controlled.

After the smoke cleared, LaBoy was temporarily placed on another unit to keep his peers from putting him in a body bag. Sunflower was an emotional wreck, but she did well disguising her feelings. She called a group to discuss what took place. Many of the youth strongly wanted LaBoy off the unit permanently. They felt he took advantage of Sunflower and the situation, because of her status as a female. They felt that if Hawkinson or Minnis were on shift that evening, LaBoy would not have acted out the way he did.

Although Sunflower knew they were right, she would never admit it in front of the youth. LaBoy was the biggest female bashing culprit, but there were others in the group who thought as he did. They had no respect for women, which was a sickness and weakness they inherited from their past environments.

*   *   *   *   *

When the group was over the youth went to their dorm rooms and prepared for bed. Sunflower went to her office to type up the incident report. Mentally, emotionally and physically drained, she sat at her desk staring at the screen. She was too tired to do anything else. She eventually mustered up enough strength to complete the paperwork. As she prepared to leave for the night, she noticed a strong stench of urine coming from the vent in her office.

Sunflower decided to do some investigating. She pulled out the flashlight from the bottom drawer of her desk and began walking around the unit. She flashed the light in areas where it was extremely dim. She checked every corner of the game room but there was nothing. She checked the corners and vents of the grand room as well. Still, she found nothing.

Sunflower entered the hallway where the small library was located. The smell of urine grew stronger. As soon as she opened the door to the library and stepped onto the throw rug in the center of the floor, she heard a sloshing sound under her feet. The stench of urine rose and met her nostrils. Sunflower's eyes began to water as she stepped back off the carpet.

She walked over and flicked on the lights. A large puddle of urine rested in the middle of the carpet. A trail of the yellow liquid led from the carpet across the tile floor to a corner of the room behind a set of bookshelves.

Sunflower cautiously walked towards the corner embracing the large flashlight as if it was a weapon. The many thoughts of a wild animal such as a raccoon or opossum camping out behind the bookshelves raced through her mind. In the past, families of raccoons had somehow managed to enter the unit from the attic up above.

She peeped around the corner. Her eyes grew wide when she spotted what lay tucked away in the corner of the room. It was a youth curled up in the fetal position sucking his thumb and sleeping away. The youth was Joby. He was saturated in urine from his waist down. Sunflower sighed deeply as she shook her head. She exited the room and went to get the third shift staff.

Whenever Joby was under extreme duress, he would always revert to his past trauma. Urinating in dark hidden places is how he coped in the past. The third shift staff was allowing him to go into the library and read until he grew sleepy. What they didn't know was that he was urinating on the carpet and in the vents of the library.

Chapter 6
Men of Distinction
Warriors of Light

The next day when Hawkinson returned from his two days off, the first thing he did as always, was read the shift summaries from the previous two days. He came across Sunflower's handwriting about the mini riot and Joby urinating in the library. Sunflower left a note specifically letting Hawkinson know that she would be in on her off day to finish the paperwork. She highlighted "off day" in bold black letters. He knew it wasn't going to be good if Sunflower was coming in on her off day.

It was an early Sunday morning and the youth were still sleeping. Hawkinson met with the rest of the team to discuss the game plan. He then posted the daily schedule before entering the hallway where the dorm rooms were. He and the rest of the team began flicking on all the lights of the dorm rooms to awaken the youth.

When the youth heard his deep soothing voice telling them it was time to get up, they prepared themselves for what lay ahead. Some of the youth were as happy as a lark to see Hawkinson. For many, he was like the father they never had. They couldn't wait to tell him about what took place while he was away for two days. He provided safety and structure in their often chaotic environment and for that they appreciated him.

Then there were the unruly, undisciplined individuals who down talked Hawkinson when he was not around. They had to prove to their peers how tough they were. Hawkinson welcomed the challenge. He knew deep down inside those were the ones that admired him the most.

After the youth completed their personal hygiene, did morning chores and attended breakfast, they returned to the grand room to attend Hawkinson's infamous Men of Distinction group. While the youth were at breakfast, Hawkinson kept Joby back to discuss his violent outburst with LaBoy and his urinating issues. Joby disclosed to Hawkinson that he lived with a foster family that had several animals, mainly dogs and cats. The many animals would urinate and defecate all over the house. The foster parents never cleaned it, so he took it as a normalized behavior. Joby explained that the dogs and cats ate better than he and his foster siblings, so in order to eat as well as them, he learned to act like them by urinating wherever he pleased. Joby was simply a product of his environment.

After processing with Joby, Hawkinson called over to the neighboring program and had LaBoy sent back over. When the other youth returned and saw LaBoy sitting in a chair before the group, they immediately frowned and began mumbling. Many slumped in their seats, which was a sign that they were refusing to participate in the group. None attempted to attack him as they did the night before when Sunflower was managing the shift. Hawkinson was on shift and the youth knew his expectations.

Sunflower walked in during the time Hawkinson was setting up for group. She observed how humble and disciplined the youth were. It was as if she stepped into the twilight zone. The sight alone infuriated her. Less than twelve hours ago, the place was a mini Beirut. She shook her head, rolled her eyes in disgust as she went to her office and heavily closed the door. Hawkinson observed her actions. Some of the youth did as well and they looked at one another and shook their heads.

Hawkinson began the group with the Men of Distinction pledge. After the pledge, he discussed how the Men of Distinction group came about. The youth that once slumped were now attentive. He explained that men of distinction are men of change. Men of distinction step up to face challenges the average person is afraid to face. Men of distinction are warriors of light. They absorb information and pass it along and above all, men of distinction are humble, respectable givers, not takers. They are renaissance men. Men of distinction are the movers, shakers, caretakers and creators of society.

Each word that bellowed from deep within Hawkinson's core and rolled off his tongue reverberated within the youths' very being. No one slept as they did in some of the other groups. No one had to go to the restroom and most of all, no one spoke out of turn. The theme of the group was, "Am I my brother's keeper?"

When Hawkinson opened the group up for questions and concerns, over three quarters of the youths' hands skyrocketed into the air. He called on the youth one at a time. They discussed their meaning of brotherhood and how it wasn't portrayed on the unit the night before. When Sunflower heard the youth discussing the situation from the past night, she exited her office and entered the grand room. She quietly stood on the outside of the group listening.

LaBoy was allowed to speak last and discuss the role he played in the violence that occurred the night before. He made up excuse after excuse for the actions he displayed. When he finished talking, Hawkinson looked him square in the eye and read him the excuses quote from his heart.

"Excuses are tools of incompetence that build monuments of nothing and those who specialize in them are seldom good at anything else. No excuses… just results." When Hawkinson finished, the entire youth committee in the grand room sat quietly as they no longer stared at LaBoy, but took a closer look at self. LaBoy lowered his head and stared at the floor.

Hawkinson asked LaBoy to stand. It was never his intention to bring shame to any of the youth, but it was his duty to address their ill intentions, just as he was about to do with LaBoy. The youth slowly stood on his feet. He hung his head as he stared at the floor. Hawkinson asked him a series of questions pertaining to the behaviors he displayed the night before. After LaBoy answered the questions to the best of his ability with no more excuses, Hawkinson approached him and placed a hand on his shoulder.

"This here is a group…a team…a band of warriors…and most importantly a family."

"This ain't my family," the youth mumbled as he continued to stare at the floor.

"It is your temporary family whether you like it or not. You have a choice to make youth LaBoy. A choice to get on board and be a changing part of what goes on around here, or a choice to return to the system where you came from. Violence, gang banging and especially disrespect of women do not live here. If you want to leave and continue those type of behaviors at your next point of destination, that is your choice. Here, we are men of distinction," Hawkinson said as he looked around the room at the other youth. "Am I my brother's keeper?" he asked the group.

"Yes I am!" the youth all responded in confident voices. Hawkinson returned his gaze to LaBoy and began speaking in a low tone to not be heard by the others.

"I've already contacted your P.O. He is calling me back soon to decide if he should send a car to get you. You broke a cardinal rule by setting off a riot with your gang affiliation. If you tell me you want to stay and put all this behind you, then you make the choice. That means all the troublesome baggage that you carry around with you has to go. This program isn't for everyone youth LaBoy. The mission statement for this treatment program is to develop youth offenders into young men who are role models. Many youth have come through here and failed miserably. Failure is what they chose. They were not yet ready. Are you ready to evolve from a boy to a young man youth LaBoy? The question is yours for the thinking. You have a little time to determine your fate. Have a seat."

Youth LaBoy was starting to perspire heavily as he sat down. Never in his life had anyone given him a choice. No one ever taught or informed him that he had the power to choose. This power to choose business was making him nervous. He never ever had to take responsibility for his actions. There was always someone to take responsibility for him. His grandma and part-time father, who only seemed to come around when the youth received his social security check, always made excuses for his ill actions.

LaBoy grew light headed. It was too much pressure placed upon him. The room seemed to spin out of control as he thought about the choices. Fear got in the way of him making a choice. Fear that others would deem him weak for turning over a new leaf, fear that word would get back to his homeboys on the street that he converted into a treatment completing choirboy. All types of fearful thoughts rushed through his mind.

Before the group was over, Hawkinson passed out journals to the youth and asked them to write how they were going to make things better. When they finished, he asked Sunflower and the other staff members if they had anything they would like to share with the group. The male rookie staff shared thoughts and gave the youth positive encouragement. When it was Sunflower's turn, she let the youth have it.

She called each youth out on the behaviors they displayed the night before. The room was silent except for the piercing words uttered from deep within Sunflower. Hawkinson observed the youth closely. Some were genuine and respected her concerns. Others hung their heads in shame. Some gritted their teeth and gave her the evil eye. It didn't matter, she wasn't the least bit intimidated. Sunflower shared what was on her mind.

When called upon, some of the youth shared concerns to Sunflower about her babysitting tactics towards some of the youth and being inconsistent with holding them accountable for their wrongdoings. As the youth continued to be speak out their concerns, Hawkinson thought back to when he constructively criticized Sunflower for the same concerns some of the youth brought to her.

Sunflower modestly accepted the concerns. Before group was over she announced the consequences the youth earned the night before. One of the consequences was no watching Sunday afternoon or Monday night professional football for a week. The majority of the youth loved football. It didn't take them long to get her message as they sat and pouted. They didn't like her decision, but they honored and respected it.

*   *   *   *   *

Hawkinson sat in his office towards the end of the shift completing paperwork when he heard a knock outside the door.

"Come in," he called out without looking up. The door swung opened and then closed rather quickly. When he looked up, Sunflower was standing on the other side of his desk with her arms folded and lips pressed tightly together. Her disposition warned him she was ready to vent.

"You okay?" he asked resting his pen.

"Hell no I'm not okay Hawk. Why is it, whenever you are off shift there is always a crisis, but as soon as you step foot in the building, the clouds part and the sun comes out? Forgive me for not being a bad ass like the almighty Hawk. I have my own style and I'm not changing. Just because I don't rule with a clad iron fist doesn't make me soft."

Hawkinson listened to his colleague vent. He knew she was just blowing off steam. He stared at her nonchalantly and allowed her to continue as he dared not interrupt.

"Today when I walked in they were all perfect little boy scouts. Last night I witnessed almost every single one of those…hellions carrying on as if this was a prison and there was a riot in the yard! Today you would think the rapture was here and everyone is waiting with golden tickets in hand for a trip to paradise! Did you know what they had the nerves to say to me? *You staff need to stop being soft and babying us. Mr. Hawkinson don't baby us. He treats us like young men!*" she said mocking the youth.

"Do you think I baby them?" she asked with her hands resting on her hips.

"I'm proud of you for the way you handled yourself out there," he said trying to avoid the question.

"Don't play spin doctor with me Hawk. I am not in the mood," she said picking up one of the stress balls on his desk and squeezing it tightly. Hawkinson took in a deep breath and slowly exhaled as he observed closely the way she squeezed the stress ball.

"Okay, yes there is some truth to what they're saying." Sunflower squinted at him as she squeezed the ball even tighter. "But hold on now," he said standing with his hands stretched out. "You could have walked out last night and never returned just like a number of staff members in the past, but you came back, on your day off. That has to account for something," he said still eyeing the ball in her hand. Hawkinson could see Sunflower's stress level slowly starting to decrease as she loosened her grip on the spherical object.

"Coming in on your off day proved to them that you do care about their wellbeing and safety. Regardless of what they said about you out there, you can't take that stuff personally, or you won't last Maya," he said in a supportive tone. Sunflower listened carefully to the words Hawkinson professed to her.

Hawkinson ventured back into his memory museum and reminded Sunflower of a time he almost walked out after being on the job two years. He remembered when just as he was about to throw in the towel after a riot jumped off during his second cycle, one of the angriest and most explosive youth approached him outside while sobbing. The youth pleaded for Hawkinson not to go. He told him he was the only staff in all the years of being in the system that ever challenged and stood up to him with tough love. After the youth finished pouring out his heart, Hawkinson wrapped an arm around his shoulder and walked the youth back inside. Hawkinson took charge of the riot and settled things down. He called a group and read the youth their rights for about an hour straight, then he listened to their concerns for about another hour. When the group was over a great deal of the youth genuinely thanked him for not giving up on them. It was at that moment, Hawkinson knew he was on to something.

Each day after that incident, Hawkinson continued to make mistakes, but he grew stronger and wiser. He paid close attention to everything. It was the youth of that cycle who nicknamed him "Hawkeyes" because they said he saw everything. It was during that cycle that a legend was born.

"I took that moment and used it to fuel my tank. My tank has been full ever since. You are the first one I ever shared this story with, and I shared it with you for a reason. If you want to walk away and not do this anymore, then fine, but don't walk away because they made you walk away. You're too good for that Maya. I have made as many mistakes as I have made good decisions with the youth. If it wasn't for my mistakes, I wouldn't have grown to be the individual I am today. The mistakes I made helped me to grow stronger," he said sitting.

"Damn it Hawk, how do you always know what to say and when to say it," she said looking away.

"Because, I say it from my heart when my heart tells me to, not really I just kind of adlib," he said humorously. Without looking at Hawkinson, Sunflower released a long frustrating sigh as she tossed the stress ball on his desk.

"I can't stand you Hawk," she said flopping down in the empty chair. She and Hawkinson discussed ways to help her maintain consistency and inner strength while working with the heavily distorted clients of Lake Apache.

When the support session was over, they both laughed it up over the stress ball Sunflower nearly squeezed to a nonexistent form.

"So are you still on for the team's Sunday evening events?" Sunflower asked.

"Wouldn't miss it for anything in the world," Hawkinson said in a jovial tone.

"Okay, hurry up and finish your paperwork so we can get out of here."

"Aye-Aye captain," Hawkinson said saluting as he sat down to complete the last of his work.

Sunday evening events involved a gathering that the staff members from Lake Apache Academy created a few cycles ago for self-care. Every Sunday during the professional football and basketball seasons, staff members from around the academy would gather at a local sports bar and grill. They would play electronic darts, pool, board games and watch the professional ball games on the many screens. Even those who didn't particularly care for sports attended. It was a time of team bonding and stress releasing.

Chapter 7
The Good Life
(A Gathering Amongst Friends)

As Hawkinson, Sunflower and the rest of the staff on the shift were leaving for the day, a few of the extra needy youth attempted to get her attention as always. She addressed them with a straight face and told them her shift was over and to bring their concerns to the staff on duty and she would speak with them when she returned to shift. One youth even had the audacity to ask her where she was going. With the same straight face and a stern tone, Sunflower told him it was not his concern and he should never address her again in that manner. For Sunflower, her new challenge was to re-establish her boundaries and remain consistent.

The youth who asked the question developed a look of confusion. He was not accustomed to Sunflower being direct and he certainly was not accustomed to her not flashing him a smile before leaving. She said good-bye to all the youth as a whole instead of the few that followed her around like lost puppies.

If Sunflower was to gain the same respect as her male counterpart, comrade, mentor and good friend, Horus Hawkinson, she was going to have to be more consistent with her boundaries. Too often in the past, Sunflower found herself being cursed out and disrespected by the youth she seemed to reach out to the most. They took advantage of her good heart and now she was taking it back. Hawkinson commended her on the good start once they exited the building.

*   *   *   *   *

Hawkinson, Sunflower and a few of their colleagues arrived at the staff gathering. The environment was live and entertaining as usual. A track by Kanye West entitled *Good Life* was playing on the jukebox.

A group of Hawkinson's comrades were huddled up together in a corner, wearing Chicago Bears jerseys and watching a Bears game. They began chanting Hawk's name as they waved him over. Life was very good for Horus Hawkinson. He looked forward to Sundays with his teammates. It was the only day of the week for them to get together and unwind from the stressful work environment.

There were plenty of laughs, good times and good eating. The staff members at Lake Apache Academy worked in a very hostile, stressful and trying environment. No one outside of their profession could ever understand what they endured on a daily basis. The sports bar and grill hosted the perfect atmosphere accompanied by the perfect theme song. As Devin Hester returned his second kick return for a touchdown, the place erupted with yelling and applauding, nearly blowing the roof off.

*   *   *   *   *

As the evening turned to nightfall, the gathering began to fizzle out. Most of Hawk's colleagues were starting to pack it in and call it a night, for it was back to the drawing board on Monday morning. Hawkinson, Sunflower and a group of their colleagues said good night to those who decided to stay a while longer and watch the Sunday night football game.

As the group of colleagues stepped outdoors, snowflakes the size of cotton balls fell rapidly from the night sky. Sunflower shivered as the frigid temperatures touched her warm face. She raised the hood on her coat and placed it over her head.

"This is why I've considered moving back to Arizona for the past few years," she told Hawkinson and the rest of her peers as they walked swiftly to their vehicles. Hawkinson knew how much Sunflower disliked the cold. He scooped up a hand full of snow, packed it together and threw it at her. She screamed out good-humoredly as the snowball hit her in the back.

"Stop playing Hawk! I knew you were going to do that!" she said laughing and screaming as she took off running all the way to her car. His colleagues joined in as they picked up snow, packed it and threw it at one another. He scooped up another hand full of the snow and formed it into an even bigger ball. He gave chase leaving the others behind while laughing it up. When Sunflower reached her car, she unlocked the door and quickly jumped in, slamming it shut behind her.

Hawkinson approached the car running. Just as he was about to throw the snowball at the window, he slipped and began a very awkward backwards fall. As he was falling, the snowball launched from his hand into the night sky. After wiping out and landing on his back, Hawkinson looked up at Sunflower who was laughing it up from the other side of the glass.

The snowball hurled back down to the earth and plopped heavily onto his face. Sunflower was really laughing it up now. Seeing her humor filled bright eyes on the other side of the glass brought a smile to Hawkinson's face. Being able to laugh at himself was something he didn't mind doing. A couple of his colleagues who were laughing hysterically helped him up. Sunflower started the engine of her car before letting the window down and handing Hawkinson a towel from her front seat.

"What just happened to you Hawk is known as karma or better yet cause and effect," Sunflower said still chuckling.

"No, it's called running too damn fast on icy pavement," he said sneezing into the towel.

"Okay, you can keep that," she said withdrawing her hands and turning up her nose. His colleagues continued to laugh it up as they brushed snow from Hawkinson's back and made fun of him. Afterwards everyone said goodnight and parted ways.

*   *   *   *   *

It was several weeks later and a few days from Thanksgiving. Every cycle the staff got together and planned a large Thanksgiving feast for the youth. Hawkinson and his teammates sat in their weekly team meeting discussing the progress of the youth and the direction of the unit as a whole. The team discussed a letter they received from the probation department concerning, Braylon Nicholson.

The judge and Braylon's probation officer wanted to give him one more chance at redeeming himself. Braylon was at the end of his rope. If he committed one more crime, which was a violation of his probation, he was going away for a long time.

The team of staff members were split on their decision for Braylon to return. One of the concerns was that he would have to start over on the yellow phase, which was one month away from being complete. Another concern was that he would be a negative influence on the other youth who were finally doing well along their treatment path. Some of the other staff felt as though he possessed leadership qualities that needed polishing.

Braylon did have leadership qualities but his stubborn attitude and anger issues were a big concern for the staff. His poor relationship with youth LaBoy Edwards who was just returning from spending two weeks in the detention center was another concern. Jimmy Minnis was the youth spokesperson. He always asked his comrades to look at things from a different angle. Maya Sunflower was the nurturer and voice of reasoning. She knew how she felt about youth Braylon, so she kept her opinion to herself. Horus Hawkinson was the disciplinarian and the voice of wisdom. He knew Braylon's return would set some of the youth off course, but ultimately that would be their test and choice to make. He voted along with the majority for the return of Braylon under strict stipulations.

The tallying of the votes revealed that most of the team wanted Braylon to return to Lake Apache Academy. It was about to get extremely interesting on unit eight. After the team meeting, one of the inexperienced counselors leaked information to one of the youth about the return of Braylon. The team's plan was to tell all of the youth about Braylon's return in a structured processing group. The one youth who had the information waited until Hawkinson, Sunflower, Minnis and the clinical staff left for the day before telling his peers. Once the information spread amongst his peers like a deadly epidemic, they set it off.

The staff on shift called Code Blue over the radio. Once again, several staff from neighboring units arrived to help restore peace and order. During the moments of chaos and confusion, a couple of the youth took off on run. They didn't get very far. They returned to the academy escorted by the local police.

*   *   *   *   *

The next day when Hawkinson arrived, he could sense that something had occurred even before the third shift supervisor had given him the report. The unit was a mess, the night chores hadn't been completed and most of the youth were still sleeping in on a school day. The energy surrounding the unit was thick and negative. Hawkinson could feel it all around him trying to penetrate his negative proof vest.

The youth who were awake sat on their beds listening to music. Some were even pacing the floor nervously when Hawkinson peered into their room. After he received the shift report, he reported the expectations of the schedule to the rest of his first shift comrades. The plan was to reintroduce the youth to Cognitively Based Treatment (CBT). Hawkinson gathered the CBT packets and placed them along with a pen on every chair in the grand room.

After the youth completed their personal hygiene and their chores, they reported to the grand room. When they walked in and viewed the packets on the chairs, many began to sigh and complain. Others eye-balled Hawkinson from across the room.

The plan was to weed out the youth who set off the unit the night before by using peer accountability. The highly motivated peers that put energy and support into the program over the course of the past few months were the first few to step up and hold the culprits accountable. CBT packets were a motivator for those that needed that extra boost to step up. They were told they didn't have to fill out the packet if they weren't involved. Choosing to take that offer, many stepped up and spoke out about their peers' disruptive behaviors.

It was disclosed that twelve youth in all set the unit off the night before, including the two that ran. Five were the main culprits and seven fed into their behaviors. After discussing the return of Braylon, Hawkinson excused the youth that came forward with the information. They returned to their daily schedule and stayed on pace with their treatment.

The culprits spent the entire morning and afternoon in group pouting and making excuses for their actions. Hawkinson wasn't buying any of what they were trying to sell. He made copies of the excuses quote and passed them out encouraging the youth to be more responsible for their actions. After wasting almost an entire shift attempting to deny and weasel their way out of the situation, the youth began filling out and internalizing the CBT packet. The two youth that attempted to run returned to the Department of Corrections that day for violating their parole.

Hawkinson and one of his colleagues spent the entire shift working diligently with the youth on their CBT packets. They had discussion after discussion about their behaviors and only took a break for mealtime, restroom and thirty minutes of recreation, which consisted of reading and drawing. Hawkinson's colleague studied the way he disciplined the youth and kept his cool the entire time. The staff member complimented Hawkinson greatly.

At the start of the next shift, Hawkinson passed the treatment baton to Minnis who made sure the youth continued to follow their restrictions. If the youth honored the restrictions and finished their packets, they would earn their way off at the end of the second shift. If the youth showed no progress, they would continue to honor the restrictions the following day.

*   *   *   *   *

Hawkinson arrived at work the next day with an optimistic outlook, but the stagnant energy warned him that some of the youth would still be on restriction. As he read the shift report from the previous two shifts, he chuckled. Sure enough, five of the ten remained on restriction. Hawkinson strapped on his invisible warrior's gear as he did every shift before entering the unit. The gear was used to defend against the negativity projected from the youth and sometimes his colleagues.

With Braylon Nicholson returning to the academy and five youth on restriction, it was sure to be an interesting shift. All the youth were up preparing for school and completing chores when Hawkinson entered the unit. Music was blaring from one of the dorm rooms, which was completely unacceptable. One of Hawkinson's expectations from the youth was social manners, which meant to greet him with a "Hello" before asking a question. There was always one or two youth that tried to test that expectation.

"Ayyyye, can I get the supply closet opened so I can get some paper towels!" one of the youth yelled at Hawkinson from down the hallway over the blaring music. Hawkinson refused to acknowledge the youth as he walked down the hallway checking and grading the dorm rooms for cleanliness.

"Aye, I said I need some paper towels so I can finish my chore!" the lanky, loud mouthed youth with very large glasses said again while looking in Hawkinson's direction. Hawkinson continued to ignore the youth. The youth stormed towards the ever so poised Hawkinson in an aggressive manner clutching the spray bottle with finger on the trigger as if it was a gun.

The majority of the youth stopped what they were doing as they focused. Some of them shook their head at the youth's foolishness. Hawkinson continued checking the rooms. He entered the youth's dorm room and turned off his music. The entire unit grew silent. Hawkinson reappeared in the hallway in the blink of an eye. Before the youth could speak, Hawkinson said good morning to him in a humble but powerful tone. Caught off guard, the youth did what he knew best. He went directly into victim mode.

"Man, why the hell you go in my room and touch my shit! That's my radio!"

"Good morning," Hawkinson said in a relaxed tone. With everyone watching, the youth continued on with his rampage. In between his vicious verbal cycle, Hawkinson slipped in a few words of advice.

"Bees don't use vinegar to catch flies... they use honey," he said looking at the supply closet. The youth stared at him while breathing heavily. Hawkinson asked Geronimo to explain the rules about the radios to his disgruntled peer.

"Radios are to only be played at a low volume when we are in our dorm rooms," Geronimo replied.

"Were you in your dorm room and was your music playing at a low volume?" Hawkinson asked the youth.

"Nope!" he answered with an attitude.

"I like music just as much as the next man. I hear it's even good for the soul, however loud music indoors on a unit of twenty-five youth just can't happen. It would be mass confusion and chaos. You have any questions or comments about the radio rule?" Hawkinson asked the youth.

"Did I lose my radio privilege?" the youth asked in an aggressive tone. Hawkinson raised one of his naturally arched eyebrows and gave the youth a peculiar look. The youth sighed heavily.

"Will twenty-four hours cover it?" the disappointed youth asked.

"Make it forty-eight and we'll call it even," Hawkinson said as he walked away and continued checking the rooms. The youth disappeared into his room grumbling and mumbling the entire time. The other youth greeted Hawkinson with a "good morning" before they bombarded him with questions and requests.

When Hawkinson looked over his shoulder, the youth that abused his radio privilege already had his boom box sitting in the hallway outside his door waiting to be collected. Hawkinson contributed the nervousness and chaos on the unit to the future return of Braylon Nicholson. The amount of influence Braylon had on his peers was incredible, even when he was absent.

*   *   *   *   *

Later that day while the youth were having lunch, the dining hall doors swung open. Sunflower and one of the rookie male staff members walked through the door followed by Braylon Nicholson. The youth of unit eight had already been instructed to have no conversation with Braylon until the introduction group. Braylon threw his hands up above his head smiling as if he was a reigning boxing champion as he strutted through the dining hall. As much as some of his peers wanted to engage, they ignored him.

Sunflower smiled at the youths' responses as she led Braylon to an empty table. When he didn't get the response he wanted from his peers, Braylon waved them off. The youth walked over to the table and sat. When he spotted Hawkinson across the room, Braylon smiled and threw his fist up above his head. Hawkinson nodded his head at the youth without smiling as he went back to monitoring the other youth.

The hair on Braylon's head was starting to grow wild and uncontrollable. The blue Department of Corrections pants sagged below his narrow waist.

The state issued shoes appeared worn. The youth looked nothing like he did when he departed. He looked unkept.

Hawkinson closely observed the behaviors of the other youth. LaBoy didn't raise his head once to acknowledge Braylon. He kept his face hidden in his plate as he ate slowly. Some of LaBoy's peers took notice in his behaviors as they chuckled and poked fun at him. Sunflower approached Hawkinson and stood next to him. The two observed the many different dynamics that were taking place.

Chapter 8
Giving Thanks Day

The dynamic duo of Hawkinson and Sunflower continued to stand together observing the youth. Every so often, Braylon would peer over at the both of them. He was secretly hoping Hawkinson would come over and welcome him back. The plan was to treat Braylon as if it was his first time at the academy.

"Do you see what I see?" Sunflower asked Hawkinson as she studied LaBoy.

"Yeah, he seems petrified. Bad move. His peers are going to eat that up," Hawkinson said. When lunch was over, all of the youth returned to the unit due to an early dismissal. It was Thanksgiving break.

The youth all sat in the grand room in the usual horseshoe setting while waiting for group to start. Braylon stood at the podium underneath the flags and pennants with his hands behind his back. As much as he tried to appear unbothered, Hawkinson watched as the youth nervously chewed on the inside of his cheek.

The introduction began. Braylon introduced himself to the group and discussed his personal treatment expectations. Afterwards each youth stood one at a time and introduced themselves to Braylon. The overall process appeared corny, but it was needed to give the returning youth a fresh start. After giving their names, his peers discussed in minor detail their position in treatment on the yellow behavioral phase. After each youth went through the introduction period, the staff took the time to introduce themselves.

Before group was over, Hawkinson and the team assigned Geronimo as Braylon's mentor. None of the other youth were to have any communication with Braylon until he passed the orientation test to re-enter the family. If he failed, he would have to wait another seventy-two hours to retake the test.

Geronimo was the perfect candidate to assist Braylon with getting back on track. He was sharp, smart and he supported Braylon the last time he was at the academy. His plan was to hold Braylon accountable while mentoring and role modeling for him. His care and concern for the scruffy looking youth ran too deep to allow him to fail.

*   *   *   *   *

Thanksgiving dinner came quickly. The youth were all dressed in their academy blazers and dress clothes. Braylon received a haircut and shave, but because he wasn't yet accepted back into the family, he wore an academy sweat suit.

Although Braylon was happy to be back at Lake Apache, he was having a difficult time adjusting to the isolation and the many stipulations placed upon him. He felt powerless. Braylon once was near the top of the treatment totem pole, now he was the last man at the bottom.

The dining hall was decorated nicely. The tables were covered with fall colored tablecloths. In the center of the tables were candy dishes filled with mints and peanuts. The color scheme of the tablecloths, balloons and ribbons hanging on the walls were chocolate brown, harvest orange and sweet corn yellow.

The youth sat at the tables socializing as they waited patiently for the serving of the meal. Braylon sat at a table all by himself. Every so often, Geronimo would venture over to his table and share small talk with him. When he would leave to go socialize with his peers, Braylon played it off as if he wasn't affected. At times, the youth looked as if he was going to break from being isolated. The treatment discipline was getting to him.

Before the meal was brought out, each youth had to express what he was thankful for and what he planned to do to help better unit eight. After all the youth shared, Braylon raised his hand high into the air. Hawkinson called upon him to speak.

"If I may, I'd like to say what I'm thankful for and what I can give back to the program to help make it better." Everyone including the staff was surprised at the appropriate choice of words and respectful tone Braylon chose to use. The youth expressed that he was thankful for not being locked up in the Department of Corrections on a very special holiday. He also expressed that he was thankful for getting a second chance at starting treatment over. Braylon expressed that he would like to help better the unit by taking on more responsibilities, such as doing all the unit chores while he was on his seventy-two hour ban from the family.

His peers applauded loudly when he volunteered to take over their chores. Some of the staff applauded as well, but not Hawkinson. He knew exactly what the crafty youth had up his sleeve. Braylon was campaigning for himself. He was trying to gain his status back at the top of the totem pole. What better way to gain it back by taking over tasks that most of his peers despised with a passion.

"Wow, that was pretty honorable of him, don't you think?" Sunflower asked humorously.

"It sounds more like running game," Hawkinson said as he observed Braylon closely.

*   *   *   *   *

Later on as everyone enjoyed the Thanksgiving Day feast, Hawkinson found his way over to Braylon's table. The hungry youth took the time to look up from the plate full of food as he bobbed his head to the jazz music playing indistinctly.

"What's going on Mr. Hawkinson? I haven't had a chance to speak with you since I've been back," he said in a cocky, overzealous tone as he patted the table for Hawkinson to sit down. Hawkinson chuckled to himself as he pulled out a chair and sat across from the youth.

"Not a lot youth Braylon, just taking notice of everyone enjoying this wonderful event, including you. Yes sir, these are some good times," he said looking around the room. "How's the food?"

"The food is good," Braylon said holding up a thumb.

"It looks good and so did you when you stood to make that speech about taking over all the chores. That was some class act," Hawkinson said as he smiled leaned forward and applauded.

"Just trying to get on track and give back Mr. Hawkinson. You know the saying, past behind and the future ahead," he said returning to his food.

"The right thing for them or the right thing for you?" Hawkinson asked looking around the room.

"The right thing for us. We're a team around here, remember," the crafty youth said shoving a spoon full of corn into his mouth.

"I just wanted to let you know that you don't owe anyone anything, but yourself."

"I know," Braylon said licking his fingers. Hawkinson handed him a napkin. The youth accepted the napkin and wiped his hands.

"No apologies, excuses or justifications for the actions that you took the last time you were here. In fact you don't even have to do their chores."

"I said I know," Braylon said with a slight tone of irritation. "I know what you're thinking Mr. Hawkinson. You think I'm trying to gain status at the top so that all my peers can look up to me as they did before."

"Is that what I'm thinking?" It sounds like you're talking about leadership."

"I ain't nobody's leader."

"Sure you are." Braylon grew silent. "You know with being a leader youth Braylon, comes a lot of responsibilities. Leadership isn't for everyone. It's not a selfish task. Leaders usually do most of the work, but rarely get any of the credit. Leadership genuinely comes from within involving ten percent of talk and ninety percent of action. Anyone can talk a good game, but very few can back it up. Are you a leader or greeder?" Braylon looked up at Hawkinson with curious eyes.

"What's a greeder?"

"A greeder is someone disguised as a leader except they want all the credit, fame and glory. Everything is about them and them only. Greeders usually have to be number one at everything all by themselves, because it makes them feel special and superficially safe. They keep a foot on everyone's throat to keep them from getting close to the top rung of the leadership ladder, fearing that they may be replaced by someone more genuine and competent. Of course, I don't see any of those greeder characteristics in you, because you're a leader, right?" Braylon shifted his eyes down to the table without responding.

"Right," Hawkinson said as he stood and smiled. "There's some pumpkin and apple pie for desert. Help yourself. Today is the national holiday for giving thanks. Thank you for sharing your time," Hawkinson said as he patted the table in a mocking manner before walking away.

Hawkinson approached the table where his colleagues were sitting. He took a seat next to Sunflower and began fixing his plate. She looked over at Braylon. He was sitting as if someone had just sucked the life force right out of him. Sunflower fixed her gaze on Hawkinson in a suspicious manner.

"Hawk, what did you do, tell the poor child he was going before a Russian firing squad?"

"I just challenged him to think about some things. I see a lot of talent in him. It'll be a shame to see it all go to waste in some jail cell or cemetery."

"It must have been some pretty serious things, because he looks like he's about to keel over." Braylon leaned back in his seat with two fingers pressed tightly to the right side of his temple. Hawkinson smiled inwardly. His mission was complete. He had tilled the soil and planted the seed of knowledge and wisdom. It was now up to Braylon to water the seed so that it may grow and prosper into fresh produce.

*   *   *   *   *

Later that evening, all of the youth except for Braylon and LaBoy went over to the complex to watch movies on the big screen. The two youth were restricted to the unit. LaBoy sat in the kitchenette area at the table with a male staff reading from the yellow phase treatment handout. As part of his contract to return to Lake Apache, the youth was on ban to all female staff campus-wide until he completed the yellow and red phase of treatment and learned to respect women.

He was behind two weeks and was desperately trying to catch up. Four more weeks and the yellow phase would be over. In all, the youth had seventeen more weeks before he could even say hello to a female.

Braylon held true to his word. He started in on the chores he promised to complete for his peers for the next seventy-two hours. The youth listened to a Stevie Wonder cd provided by Hawkinson as he worked diligently. He swept and mopped floors. He wiped down the furniture. He cleaned the fish tank, windows and took out the trash. He even cleaned all the restrooms on the dorm wing, which was a task no one wanted.

When Hawkinson would exit his office to go to the copier, he noticed Braylon from his peripheral watching him. When he focused in on the youth, Braylon quickly looked away and continued working. Hawkinson chuckled to himself as he returned to his office.

Some time later, there was a knock at Hawkinson's door. When he looked up Braylon was standing at the door. The youth appeared exhausted as he wiped perspiration from his brow.

"Youth Braylon, how can I help you sir?"

"You have any trash that needs emptied?" he asked refusing eye contact. Hawkinson stood and pulled the trash basket from underneath his desk and walked it over to Braylon who was still refusing eye contact. The youth accepted the trash and emptied it into a large plastic garbage can.

"Is that it?" he asked still refusing eye contact.

"That's it in here. Did you check with Ms. Sunflower and the other staff?"

"No," he mumbled. Hawkinson picked up the phone and called Sunflower. After she answered the call, he sent Braylon down to her office to get the trash.

"Hey youth Braylon, good job out there cleaning. It hasn't smelled this fresh around here in awhile. Your work doesn't go unnoticed," Hawkinson said giving the youth encouragement.

"Thanks," Braylon said as he pulled the garbage can out of the office. The chipped tooth youth looked over his shoulder and gave Hawkinson a genuine half smile before walking away. The chipped tooth made him look like an innocent young boy. Hawkinson smiled to himself as he went back to work.

*   *   *   *   *

It was the final day of Braylon's ban to his peers. It was also the final day of him completing everyone's chores, which was starting to wear on the youth. It seemed like he cleaned from the time he got up until it was time for bed. The youth was also getting cabin fever. Watching his peers go over to the complex for sports and other entertainment over the Thanksgiving weekend was getting to him.

It was Sunday morning after breakfast and the youth were on their way to the complex for a game of indoor flag football, something Braylon enjoyed almost as much as playing basketball. He was restricted from going due to his ban from interacting with his peers; however, the ban would be over later that evening before bedtime.

Braylon immediately began to regress and cycle into a pattern of his old behaviors. It started with the muscles in his lower jaw moving up and down, negative self-talk and pacing back and forth. The peers that were in corrections with him knew what was coming next when they noticed the movement of his lower jaw. They stayed clear of his path. Geronimo approached and tried to talk to him. The frustrated Braylon cursed Geronimo. He backed off. The more Braylon spoke negatively to himself, the angrier he became.

When the staff approached him to process, the youth verbally exploded in sporadic sequences. Braylon had it fixed in his thoughts that if he wasn't going to the complex, no one was going. He sabotaged the event by physically acting out.

The youth found nearby cleaning supplies and began dumping them all over the floor. He walked into his peers' rooms randomly and took things that didn't belong to him. Minnis approached and attempted to process with him, but the persistent youth ignored him as well.

Hawkinson was radioed to the scene. He approached and surveyed the area. It was as if a preschooler had thrown a tantrum. Things were everywhere. Braylon was walking around with his chest expanded looking for more things to destroy. Hawkinson stood in his path. The youth retreated and went the opposite direction, looking over his shoulder the entire time.

He disappeared around a corner. Hawkinson and Minnis followed him. They heard the sound of brooms and mops crashing to the floor.

By the time they reached Braylon, he was holding a five-gallon bucket of laundry detergent.

"If you come any closer, I swear on my momma I'll dump this shit all over the floor," he said with a straight face. Minnis asked the youth to put the bucket down. Hawkinson stood observing the youth who refused eye contact with him. More male staff arrived. Hawkinson held up a hand signaling for them to hold their positions.

"Where is this going to get you youth Braylon?" Minnis asked. The youth ignored him as his eyes darted back and forth as if he was searching for something. Minnis cautiously approached as he slowly held out his hand.

"Put it down and let's go talk about this," he told Braylon.

"I don't want to talk," he yelled as he continued to search the area. Minnis slowly put his hand on the handle of the bucket. Braylon snatched the bucket away as he bolted past both staff running awkwardly with the bucket. He then turned to face the men and began dumping the liquid soap all over the tile floor.

"Come get some!" he yelled repeatedly. As the staff approached him from the other end, Braylon quickly spun around and began dumping soap on the floor inviting them to come and get him as well. One staff member had gotten too close to the soap and slipped. He wiped out and crashed hard to the floor.

Braylon threw the bucket to the floor and bolted into one of the rooms. By the time Hawkinson, Minnis and the other staff reached the room, Braylon had wedged himself in the corner behind the wardrobe closet. The behaviors were bizarre for a teenager, but not for a youth who'd been locked up behind bars since he was twelve years old.

Braylon never had a chance to grow and mature. Cognitively and emotionally he was a young child. The issues he harbored grew and festered. It was unfortunate to watch a young adult going through such a behavioral cycle. Braylon and Hawkinson peered at one another through a space between the wall and the wardrobe.

Hawkinson caught a bird's eye view of the emotions that interchanged on the youth's face as he hid behind the wardrobe. At that moment, Braylon wasn't the tough street kid he wanted everyone to believe he was. He was a hurt young child that needed a lot of healing. Hawkinson asked everyone to step out of the room. There was some hesitation, but trusting the call of their senior leader, the staff stepped out of the room into the hallway.

Hawkinson leaned up against the wardrobe and silenced himself. This went on for some time. The silence made Braylon uncomfortable as it did most people. Eventually there was some movement on the other side of the wardrobe. The youth slowly stepped out and sat on the window seal.

Hawkinson remained silent. Silence was golden in his book. It was the best medicine and solution to most conflicting problems.

"I guess I messed up, huh," Braylon said looking down at the floor.

"Do you think you messed up?" Hawkinson asked.

"See what y'all made me do. None of this would have happened had you just let me go to the complex."

"So what you're saying is all we have to do is give you what you want when you want it and you'll comply. Sounds like an offender's mentality."

"I'm saying all they had to do was let me go and we wouldn't be here dealing with this."

"We're here dealing with this because your ignition switch doesn't work in your cognitive functioning. You can't handle the word *no*. No doesn't mean forever in some cases, it's just for the time being. If you don't learn how to accept the word no, your life is going to be one big disappointment." Braylon sat quietly listening at first. What Hawkinson was saying made sense, that is until the little man inside began telling Braylon not to trust Hawkinson, because he'll disappoint him just like everyone else. He told Hawk that he might as well stop talking because his mind was made up and he was going to do whatever he wanted.

Hawkinson didn't debate him. He knew Braylon was having a debate with the little person inside. Just like most people who'd been hurt at a young age, Braylon possessed a little person inside. The little person spawned from the child who never matured internally with the rest of its physical body. The little person inside would step up and challenge anyone who set off its intruder alarm. Whenever the little person felt challenged, threatened or misunderstood it would argue and fight anything and anyone in its path.

Hawkinson knew the best cure for the little person inside was to give it space and approach it cautiously so that it could recover without feeling threatened. After about an hour of silence, the little person inside of Braylon shrank and went into hiding. The sixteen-year old remorseful Braylon spoke up and agreed to clean up the mess he made. Minnis gave Hawkinson the thumbs up.

"I respect your patience Hawk. He's going to be a tough one," Minnis said walking away scratching his head.

"Yes he is, but we've been down this road many times before," Hawkinson said as he supervised the youth cleaning up the mess.

Chapter 9
Phase Two
(The Red Phase)

As time passed, Braylon continued to struggle with adapting to his new role at the bottom of the totem pole. His peers looked at him differently after the soap on the floor incident and destruction of their property. Braylon definitely lost some cool points. Even the emotionally challenged youth were labeling Braylon as a pressure case.

The term pressure case was a word used by the youth from the Department of Corrections to describe someone who was mentally or emotionally unstable and cracked under pressure. Braylon wasn't a pressure case. He just simply hadn't been challenged cognitively the way he had before arriving at Lake Apache. He was used to roaming freely causing chaos and wreaking havoc wherever he resided. What Braylon was going through was normal. He was getting the reality check of his life.

Hours turned into days, and days turned into weeks. Creation or time as most people call it was speeding along. The yellow phase was nearing an end and the red phase was on the horizon.

Those who did not successfully complete the yellow phase were at risk of becoming a holdover. Braylon was one of the youth at risk along with Joby Kiddwell and a hand full of others. Geronimo Coltrane had been spending a great deal of his time working with Braylon, but the stubborn youth was burning him out.

Geronimo met with Hawkinson and the rest of the team of staff to ask if he could relinquish his duties as Braylon's mentor. He felt as though he was putting too much energy into Braylon and not enough into himself. Geronimo was in jeopardy of not making the red phase if he did not complete his last two anger management assignments. Hawkinson always taught the youth to speak up when stumped with an issue.

The staff members granted Geronimo his request. He was no longer Braylon's mentor. Hawkinson, Minnis, Sunflower and a couple of other staff stepped up and took over the duty. Braylon wasn't too thrilled. He knew Hawkinson and company wasn't going to play his manipulating games.

Braylon was sure to be a holdover during the next cycle. He was too far behind. He had two out of eleven assignments done on the yellow phase with only one week remaining before the red phase began. No youth in the history of Lake Apache ever bounced back and graduated after being that far behind.

*   *   *   *   *

It was two days before Christmas. Hawkinson sat in his office with the two family therapists, finalizing the treatment assignments for the red phase. There was a knock at his door. When he looked up, Braylon was standing at the door holding a stack of disorganized treatment papers. Hawkinson waved him in and pointed to an empty chair as he continued working closely with the family therapists.

The youth crossed the threshold looking around at the decorated office. He slowly and carefully sat down in a chair on the side of Hawkinson's desk. Hawkinson and the therapists conversed a little while longer before they included Braylon in the conversation.

The therapist asked the youth detailed questions about his family. The purpose of the questions was to get family members involved in the youth's treatment as a support. An outside support team would benefit the youth's transition back into society.

Braylon avoided the questions about his family. Realizing he wasn't ready to venture into that realm of treatment, the therapists backed off. After the therapists left the office, Braylon sat quietly in the chair shuffling through his paperwork.

"Youth Braylon, what can I do for you?"

"I need some help on these treatment assignments," he said looking down at the disheveled papers.

"I have a few minutes, let's see what you have."

"A few minutes, this is going to take longer than a few minutes," he said looking up at Hawkinson.

"Then it's going to have to wait until tomorrow morning. I have a game to coach tonight. Besides, had you showed up at your regularly scheduled session we wouldn't be having this discussion."

"I was at the gym. Why didn't you come get me?"

"This is your treatment, not mine. It's not my responsibility to come get you. Besides, I told you the time of your session before you went to the gym, but yet you still chose to go play ball. Get your priorities in order sir." The youth sighed deeply as he slumped in his chair and waved Hawkinson off.

"Is that how you feel?" Hawkinson asked. The frustrated youth refused to respond as he stared at the floor.

"You have fifteen minutes to work on your assignments with me before I leave," Hawkinson said before writing in his weekly planner. Silence became the youth's theme. He sat quietly grinding the muscles in his lower cheek. Hawkinson used a therapy technique on Braylon known as planned ignoring. Sunflower approached the door.

"Are you in a session?" she asked.

"Apparently not," he responded looking at the slumping youth. Sunflower asked Hawkinson a couple of questions about a treatment plan for another youth while Braylon sat and pouted as time ticked away. The youth mumbled something under his breath.

"Excuse me youth Braylon, you have something you want to share?" Hawkinson asked.

"I said I'm tired of people trying to play me."

"Are you referring to anyone in particular?" Hawkinson asked.

"I'm referring to whoever is listening," he shot back.

"I think I'll be leaving now," Sunflower said as she gave Hawkinson the thumbs up for good luck before walking away.

"Are you ready to talk now?"

"I'm talking, ain't I?"

"I guess you are. Who's trying to play you youth Braylon?"

"These punk ass kids around here, my family and these lame as staff," he said popping his knuckles.

"Am I one of the lame ass staff who's trying to play you?"

"Come on man don't be using those treatment mind tricks on me like I'm stupid."

"I have no tricks and I definitely don't think you're stupid. I'm simply asking a question." Braylon sighed deeply and shook his head.

"All of my peers are mad at me. Geronimo don't want to be my mentor. The other staff treat me like I'm invisible, and you're trying to get out of having a session with me so you can go coach some ol' stupid game. I might as well go back to D.O.C."

"Is the Department of Corrections where you want to be?"

"It's easier than being here. I can lay in my bunk in my cell and watch t.v. all day."

"So why did you come back if your life was so good there?" Braylon grew quiet before answering.

"I thought things would be different."

"I thought they were."

"This is not the kind of different I was expecting." Hawkinson's timer on his desk went off. Braylon looked at the timer. "What's that?" he asked.

"Time is up. I have to go. We'll pick this up tomorrow." Braylon sat quietly in his chair as Hawkinson stood up and put his laptop in his bag. He walked over and removed his coat from the coat rack.

"That's what I'm talking about. This is some bull," Braylon mumbled as he stood.

"I have a few words of advice for you youth Braylon. Find out what's important to you and make it your first priority. If you don't like the way things are going in your life, do something positively constructive to change it. I'll see you tomorrow," Hawkinson said as he picked up his bag and threw it over his shoulder.

"Right," the disappointed youth said as he gathered his disheveled papers and strolled out of the office grinding his jaw. Hawkinson stopped by all the offices and said goodnight to his colleagues as he always did. He stopped by Sunflower's office and knocked on the open door.

"Hey," she said looking up from the computer monitor.

"Hey, keep an eye on youth Braylon. I have a feeling he may bolt."

"Did he say he felt like running?"

"No, but I just want us to be cautious. He's a little emotionally unstable at this time."

"He's not going anywhere Hawk. Youth Braylon is throwing a fit because his favorite staff, *mister the sun is always shining,* isn't giving him the attention he wants," Sunflower said returning to her computer monitor. Hawkinson said goodnight before exiting the office. As he walked through the unit, he took notice of his surroundings. Braylon was sitting in the back of the television room with his hood over his head. Thadius Powers, the most gentle, quiet, observant youth Hawkinson had ever known, sat right in front of the television as he did everyday. He stared at the television without blinking. It was a routine Powers developed since arriving to the academy.

Geronimo and a few of the other coordinators approached Hawkinson and asked if they could have a coordinators meeting some time in the near future. Hawkinson agreed to have the meeting while at the same time observing a few of the youth in a corner looking suspicious.

He walked towards the youth in the corner. They sat up straight as an arrow when they noticed him coming. As he approached, Hawkinson noticed a shirt spread out on the floor. The youth all looked away as if they knew nothing about the shirt. Hawkinson held out his hand. The youth continued to ignore him. He cleared his throat. One of the youth tapped another on the arm. The youth dug deep down into his pocket and retrieved a set of dice. He placed them in Hawkinson's hand. The persistent Hawkinson cleared his throat again. The youth sighed deeply as he dug into his opposite pocket and retrieved another set of dice.

Hawkinson gave all three youth a writing assignment on in house gambling which was a major restriction. He slipped the dice in his pocket and shook his head before walking away. Hawkinson smiled internally at the intelligence the youth displayed by using the shirt to silence the dice when they rolled them. The youth were gambling with their late evening snacks, which was sad but even funnier to Hawkinson.

*   *   *   *   *

When Hawkinson reached the outdoors, a fresh crop of snow covered the ground. Purple streaks of light flashed across the sky illuminating his surroundings. Hawkinson took notice and looked down at the ground. Large animal footprints covered the area. There were many of them. Hawkinson followed the footprints out to the parking lot. He stood next to his vehicle and used his eyes to continue following the prints. He followed the prints out near the opening of the woods. When he looked up from the prints, his eyes met the yellow glowing eyes of several coyote.

The coyote stared at Hawkinson as he stared at them in return. The largest of the coyote stepped out from the pack. He stared at Hawkinson a little while longer before throwing his head back and howling at the bright pumpkin orange moon rising high in the Northeast.

When the coyote finished howling it lowered its head and continued staring at Hawkinson. The rest of the pack threw their heads back and let out a long howl. When they finished howling, the leader of the pack raised his hind leg and marked its territory by urinating. It stared at Hawkinson a while longer before breaking its gaze and dashing off into the woods with the rest of the pack on its heels.

Hawkinson surveyed the area for more of the coyotes before getting into his car. He pulled out his cell phone and called the unit warning all the staff to be on alert for coyote in the area. In all of his years of working at

Lake Apache, Hawkinson had never known any coyote to venture onto the campus. He had always seen them on the country roads, but never in the residential areas. The global climate was changing. The earth's megahertz had risen from eight to twelve in the past several years, which meant global change was affecting everything from the weather to animals and human behavior.

*   *   *   *   *

Christmas Day had come. Most of the youth were grateful for the gifts they received, but then there were those few who always felt as if they did not get enough. Hawkinson and his colleagues held a group with the youth on entitlement issues and possessiveness. He tied the two characteristics into the youths' offending behaviors that landed them in the system.

Most of the youth walked away from the group having learned a great lesson, but then there were those few who did not seem phased by the message of the powerful group. They continued to display ungrateful attitudes. Youth Geronimo, Brennen and a few other peers attempted to talk to the ungrateful youth also known as system babies. System babies were children that grew up in the juvenile system and were used to everything being handed to them. They proved to be the most ungrateful youth of all.

*   *   *   *   *

As time went on, Hawkinson continued his individual sessions with Braylon. The new year had come and gone. Braylon was starting to make some effort and take responsibility for his scheduled sessions. When his peers went to the complex for sports, Braylon opted to stay back for therapy sessions with Hawkinson. Even when he wasn't scheduled for a session, Braylon would stay back and work on assignments. He was trying his best to play catch up. The red phase had begun, but Braylon was still stuck in the midst of the yellow phase.

Many of the other youth began observing the changes in Braylon. His power and control issues began to decrease. His episodes of physical aggression decreased and he developed a more positive attitude that was noticed by others around the campus. The staff from other units appreciated the youth's efforts and they commended him.

Sunflower approached Hawkinson's door and knocked before entering. She was smiling and shaking her head.

"What did I do this time?" he asked noticing the smile.

"You've started something around here with your one on one session with youth Braylon."

"What do you mean?"

"I was facilitating my life skills group with the youth and half of them shared that they want to have one on one sessions with you. The same kind of session you're having with youth Braylon. They said if you can change him, you can change anyone," she said still smiling.

"Why are you smiling like that?"

"Because I think that is a great compliment to what you do around here. Even youth Powers, who does nothing but watch television and stare at me through the lenses of those eerie glasses voiced his opinion about wanting to meet with you. I don't know Hawk. I think you might be in over your head," she said walking away. Sure enough when Hawkinson exited his office and entered the milieu, a group of the struggling youth approached him, even Thadius Powers who hadn't said all of two words to him prior to that moment. They asked if they could meet with him for a session to work on yellow phase treatment issues.

Hawkinson never denied any of the youth an individual session, but at the same time he never allowed himself to out work the client. He came up with a proposal. The youth had to give up their recreation time and video game time in exchange for individual session time. The youth that were serious about their success in treatment agreed to the proposal. They even signed off on the proposal. The youth who were not as serious about their treatment backed off and refused to sign an agreement or give up their video game time.

Hawkinson did not force the issue. He allowed the youth to make their own decision when it came to treatment. He wasn't doing treatment for them, they were doing it for themselves. Some of the youth evolved differently than others. Some approached treatment the way some people approach life, with the attitude of success.

*   *   *   *   *

It was early evening when Hawkinson decided to wrap things up for the day. The second part of his day was about to begin with mentoring sessions for struggling teens and later he'd have basketball practice with a group of fired up children ages 8 through 10. A group of other staff including Sunflower, were leaving as well.

It was unspoken but apparent that everyone was looking out for coyote once they went outdoors and walked to their vehicles. No one conversed. Their eyes focused on the wood line next to the parking lot. The only noise that penetrated the silence surrounding the darkness was the crunching sound of snow underneath their feet.

Once they reached the parking lot successfully, everyone breathed a sigh of relief except for Hawkinson who seemed unphased by the emergence of the coyote. He popped his trunk and removed a snowbrush as he began cleaning the fresh fallen snow from his windows. The other staff warmed their automobiles as they brushed snow away from their windshields as well.

"Hey Hawk, there's a group of us going bowling tonight. Would you like to join us?" Sunflower asked as she brushed snow from her windshield.

"I'd like to, but I have a full slate. I have a mentoring session with a couple of teens."

"How about afterwards?" she asked.

"I have basketball practice with a group of energetic eight to ten year olds. We have a big game this Friday night. I have to get them prepared."

"Do you ever take time for yourself and live a little?" she asked.

"Yep, every morning after I wake. When most of the world is dead asleep I'm either running, working out, reading or having quiet time to reflect on my future goals. I call it the good life."

"I applaud you for your ambition and drive Hawk. Howerver, the good life is also about having a laugh or two while fellowshiping with friends."

"She's right Hawk," another one of his colleagues cleaning off his vehicle responded. Hawkinson thought about Sunflowers comment.

"Okay, maybe when the basketball season is over in a few weeks, I'll have to take you guys up on that offer. I guess I can dust off my ball and break out the golden shoes. I hope you've overcome that condition you have," he said to Sunflower as he tossed the snowbrush inside the trunk before slamming it shut.

"What condition are you referring to Hawk?"

"The sore loser condition."

"Hawk, since when have you known me to be a sore loser?" He looked up at the heavens as he began filling Maya in on all the times she displayed the condition of being a sore loser.

"Wow, you sound bitter. Are you still holding on to that?" she asked with a hint of sarcasm.

"You bring a whole different meaning to the definition of sore loser. If one was to look up sore loser in the dictionary there would be a disgruntled mug shot of you posing very sorely," he said with a disgruntled crazed look as he shimmied around. His colleagues in the parking lot laughed at Hawkinson's antics.

"Okay Hawk, you're not in group talking to the youth so you can stop with the old shimmy-shimmy coco pop dance routine," Sunflower said mocking Hawkinson's shimmy from the shoulders routine. Their colleagues laughed it up as they enjoyed the feud. He tried his best to not laugh, but he just couldn't refrain. Sunflower had him summed up.

"You see, I got this here sore loser thing all figured out," she said deepening her voice. "I got eleven notches of working with troubled teens on my belt to prove it," she said shimmying from side to side. Their colleagues continued to laugh it up as Sunflower imitated Hawkinson to perfection.

"Okay, okay you win. You're not a sore loser, just a poor imitator," he said raising his hands as if to surrender.

"You know what they say, mockery is the first form of flattery."

"Well in that case I am truly flattered, Hawk. Don't let the kids show you up at practice tonight. I don't want to hear about how sore you are all day tomorrow," Sunflower said walking towards her car.

"I don't complain. I just express my feelings. Drive safely everyone. I heard we're supposed to get six to ten inches of more snow accompanied by blustery cold winds," Hawkinson said.

"Please, no more winter blues. It's only January and I'm sick of it already. As we speak I am definitely in my imagination basking under the warm rays of the Arizona sun," said Sunflower.

"It sounds like you need a little summertime," Hawk said as he reached into his car and pressed play on the cd player. The smooth sounds of *Summertime*, by Will Smith aka the Fresh Prince and Jazzy Jeff filtered through the speakers and soared out into the airwaves. Some of the staff began pumping their fists and rejoicing as they continued to brush snow from their vehicles. For the next five minutes, Hawkinson transformed a cold snowy winter's late January evening into a fun, hot summer July day. Everyone including Sunflower stuck around just to hear the spirit raising sounds of *Summertime,* that seemed to instantly warm up the atmosphere and break the monotony of the frigid winter blues.

Chapter 10

B.E.L.I.E.V.E.

(Best Ever Living Individual Evolving Very Excellently)

Hawkinson met with two young foster teens for a mentoring session. One of the teens was struggling in school with disciplinarian issues. The other teen was struggling with curfew and peer pressure, which was affecting him in every aspect of his young life; however, their behaviors compared nothing to the behaviors of the teens at Lake Apache that Hawkinson counseled on a daily basis.

One at a time, the teens zoomed in on Hawkinson's conversation as he shared his input on ways to support them. The teens weren't always attentive. At the beginning of the sessions, it took time for them to get to know Hawkinson before they could trust him with their innermost thoughts and past issues.

After Hawkinson passed the teens' trust test, they inducted him into their hall of shame. Hawkinson would tour with them as they traveled through the halls of their memory museums, sharing with him their most fragile memories, something Hawkinson viewed as very sacred. Hawkinson and the foster mother, who was stupendous at her duties of raising the two teens in addition to her own two children, filled a void in the two teens life. Hawkinson respected her greatly for being the guiding light in their lives.

Back in the fall, the younger of the two teens invited Hawkinson to his homecoming football game, which he accepted the invitation with honors.

What the teen didn't know was that Hawkinson was asked to stand in as a role model and mentor for him during the halftime presentation, which honored the parents of the football players.

When the teen approached the center of the field expecting to greet his foster mother, but instead was greeted by Hawkinson, his eyes displayed confusion. The confusion was quickly replaced with excitement, delight and pride. He shared an embrace with Hawkinson before honoring him with a team souvenir cup and team button pin. The experience would forever hang on the walls in the teen's memory museum as well as Hawkinson's.

*   *   *   *   *

Later that evening after the mentoring sessions, Hawkinson traveled to the gym for a late evening basketball practice with a co-ed team of children. Hawkinson and his trusty assistant coach conducted the practice with extreme structure and focus. The young boys and girls learned more than just the fundamentals of basketball. They learned how to compete with enthused passion while displaying sportsmanship. They also learned how to work as a team, but most importantly, they learned how to believe.

B.E.L.I.E.V.E was an acronym Hawkinson came up with that stood for Best Ever Living Individual Evolving Very Excellently. Hawkinson taught and coached every child under his umbrella that very philosophy. One of the most important things for any child was to believe they are the best at what they do. Believing in themselves made way for self esteem. He hoped it would encourage them to carry a positive, healthy attitude over to their young adult life.

Hawkinson had a deep admiration for the parents who involved themselves in their children's progression throughout the season by attending their practices and games. It showed a sense of commitment, honor, involvement and love for their children. That meant everything to Hawkinson, especially considering he was surrounded daily by youth who had no one actively committed and involved in their lives.

*   *   *   *   *

It was the end of the week, which meant Friday night games. Hawkinson and his assistant coach corralled the children together as they prepared them for another learning session of healthy fun team competition. Each week he designated one of the children as team captain. It gave the children a chance to learn readiness and leadership.

Leadership for the children meant developing courage, confidence, responsibility and a sense of self-worth. Readiness prepared the children mentally and physically for any unexpected experience or action. The children loved the challenge. Hawkinson always searched for the spark of light in the children's eyes to help him determine who was ready to be team captain. When the light was spotted, he knew who was ready.

Defense, boxing out, team unity and shot selection is what Hawkinson engraved in the children's thought process all week during practice. When it was game time, he asked them to repeat back to him the mission. The children were able to do so word for word without any hesitation.

During the huddle up just before opening tip off, the children stacked their hands upon one another. The energy pulsating from them was electrifying. The team captain led the count from one thru three. The children all threw their hands up and yelled out B.E.L.I.E.V.E., nearly blowing the roof off the gymnasium.

Hawkinson studied the environment before tip off. The gymnasium was packed. There was standing room only. All eyes were on center court. It was the game of the season. It was the tale of two hard working well coached undefeated teams going head to head. The word all week was that the other team had more superior athletes with speed and height, but Hawkinson knew they didn't have what his team had— the unseen force of believing.

The other team appeared quicker and they jumped higher. They ran faster and they had a big kid that Hawkinson coached the previous fall who dominated the middle position. Hawkinson had two leaders on his team with a tenacious defensive stance. Because, he coached both children for the past five years and knew exactly what they were capable of achieving, his confidence in them soared.

Their defensive skills were good, but that night they stepped up to the challenge and showed greatness, which made their teammates great as well. They executed the defense assignment flawlessly. It was an overall team effort as Hawkinson's team dominated defensively the entire game.

Late in the game the other team stormed back by scoring three straight baskets to take the lead by one. With seventeen seconds to go, Hawkinson's team tied the game on a free throw. The other team drove the ball down and put up a shot. They missed. Hawkinson's team boxed out, snatched the rebound and dribbled the ball up the court with nine seconds left in the game.

The team captain dribbled the ball up the court to the right side of the lane and pulled up a jumper with just seconds to go. The ball banked off the backboard and rolled off the rim. Hawkinson's team captured the offensive rebound and Put the ball up, only to have the round ball awkwardly bounce off the other side of the rim. Time expired and the game was over.

There was no overtime in this particular league, which meant the game ended in a defensive 10 to 10 tie. It was one of the greatest defensive games ever played and coached. No one lost and everyone won including the families and friends of the children that showed up to cheer them on. The sportsmanship between both teams at the end of the game was phenomenal. The children and coaches shook hands and congratulated one another. It was a picture perfect moment of what the league stood for, great sportsmanship and healthy team competition.

Fans, parents, grandparents and others approached Hawkinson and his assistant coach at the end of the game. They congratulated the two coaches and expressed how well of a job they have done all season. Hawkinson thanked everyone graciously before approaching the child he formerly coached from the other team. He showed him love by giving him a hug and congratulating him for having an outstanding game and for leading his team back with the three big shots in the clutch.

Hawkinson defined love as a deep feeling of affection and care and concern toward a person from that which arises from a sense of oneness. He defined a deed as a praiseworthy action that is carried out. Everyone according to Hawk was a part of oneness. The actions that were worth high praise for the children he coached, mentored and counseled were out of care and concern from a sense of oneness. The actions displayed were loving deeds for the children by a man called Hawk.

*   *   *   *   *

That following Sunday morning Hawkinson facilitated the Men of Distinction group. The topic of this particular group was entitled "Emotional Expressions". Treatment for many of the youth had taken a quantum leap forward. They were now on the red phase, which meant things were about to evolve. The youth were entering the anger danger zone, which meant they were about to get heavy into expressing emotions brought up by the phantoms and demons of their past. Hawkinson and his colleagues entered the red phase under extreme caution.

The youth struggled greatly with openly expressing themselves during the start of the group. Many of them journaled their emotions in their journals while others played the Billy Bad Ass and Tough Tony roles. In their cognitively distorted thought processes, playing the roles kept them in control and from becoming emotionally exposed.

Playing the tough role only made matters worse. The tougher the youth acted, the more they came undone at the core fabric of their emotions. Hawkinson therapeutically challenged the youth. When they couldn't handle his cool calm cognitive approach, they shifted the focus on one another and launched verbal threats.

The "Emotional Expressions" group would have appeared unsuccessful to the average person who would have been a guest sitting outside the group looking in, but group was a success. Emotions were flying high. It was just as Hawkinson predicted. If the youth displayed no emotions, the group would have been unsuccessful. Emotions allowed the youth to get in touch with feelings. By getting in touch with their feelings, the youth allowed themselves to experience something real, something to help them heal.

*   *   *   *   *

As time progressed, the Emotional Expression Group evolved. The youth began to settle into the group and express themselves in a more appropriate manner. Youth Geronimo was the group's co-facilitator. He earned the position due to his dedication and advancement in treatment.

As a group leader, his assignment was to research and define the term emotion. Once found, he described emotion as a mental energy set in motion through feelings such as joy, grief, fear, hate and love. He went on to express that in a balanced healthy person, emotions are managed by the intellect. Unhealthy, unmanaged emotion produces chaos and unstability. Unexpressed it produces confusion and conflict. Bottled up like sealed cola, it creates extreme pressure exploding and causing internal and external damage to the human physical structure.

As the group continued to evolve, Hawkinson would play a variety of different music as he encouraged the youth to journal how the song affected them emotionally. One of the the songs was by Knarles Barkley, entitled *Crazy*. The youth allowed the music to move them as they later recorded the feelings in their journal. The severly emotionally challenged youth rocked back and forth. They closed their eyes to fight the pain of their emotions and feelings.

When the group was over there was a period of silence on the unit. Many of the youth had slipped into a mild state of depression as they ventured into deep thought with the emotional phantoms resurrected from the graveyards of their subconscious. Treatment was starting to deepen.

*   *   *   *   *

Braylon and the other youth on the yellow phase continued to meet with Hawkinson in a small group. Some were itching to advance to the red phase, while others displayed fear of advancement. The fear spawned from having to express their emotions in the group before others.

Expressing emotions and feelings was unheard of in the environments from which Braylon and his peers derived. They preferred to face physical confrontations rather than discuss their feelings openly in an individual session, let alone in a group. Some stated they would rather take their locked down emotions to the grave with them. Unfortunately, that wasn't an option. In order to advance from the red phase to the blue phase, the youth had to bypass the most dreaded group of them all, Emotional Expressions.

One evening during an Emotional Expressions group, one of the more angry youth began to express his hidden feelings. He expressed that he hated the very skin that covered his bones. He hated the bones that made up his physical structure. He hated the evil within that imprisoned his spirit. He began to discuss all the horrific things he'd done to others. Some were people he knew and others were complete strangers.

The youth had everyone's undivided attention. The deeper he went into his closet and drug out the skeletons, the more he began to transform into a different individual. The frown in his brow dissolved away. The complexion of life returned to his flesh. The darkness in the pupil of his eyes brightened.

Tears streamed from his ducts like water streaming from a frozen brook on the first warm day of spring. When the youth finished processing and sharing his feelings, he'd sunk so deep into his chair that he was barely visible.

His peers applauded his courageous efforts. The youth sat with his head hung. Hawkinson sat back observing the group and from his observation he gathered that there wasn't a selfish motive in the room. Despite the many horrendous behaviors the youth displayed and the crimes they committed in their past, Hawkinson learned that they had compassion and a heart.

Hawkinson instructed the youth to record their emotions from the group in their journals. He pressed the play button on the cd player. The soulful sounds of Earth Wind and Fire's, *Devotion* infiltrated through the speakers. The youth began writing as Phillip Bailey's lyrics filled the airwaves. The definition of Devotion is the act of private worship. The youth welcomed the private worship. They listened to Phillip Bailey and the rest of Earth, Wind and Fire in silence as they recorded their innermost feelings.

*   *   *   *   *

As time lapsed, some of the youth on the red phase began to relapse. They descended to a place in their emotions that felt familiar and comfortable, a place called the escape route. Cognitively, there was no challenge or struggle when the youth blocked themselves from feeling emotions. They resorted back to foul language and uncontrollable behaviors, not concerned about the consequences and repercussions of their actions.

It was an expectation in the treatment world for youth to regress and relapse. They were entering a part of treatment that was challenging. The question was how far back would they regress? Regression was normal for anyone going through a treatment program. Surprisingly for the first time in the history of Hawkinson's career, none of the youth regressed so far back that they couldn't recover.

Hawkinson and Minnis were amazed at the response of the youth, so amazed that Minnis came up with a plan. Instead of just adding music to the youths' treatment, he thought it would be more healing and helpful if the youth performed their favorite style of music, while incorporating it into the red phase of treatment.

There were many genres of music including jazz, positive rap, country, hard rock, soft rock, rhythm & blues and gospel. The youth were very diverse in the musical realm. Minnis knew it was going to be a challenge, but he took on the challenge as he often did when it came to supporting the youths' success in treatment.

*   *   *   *   *

Things began a little rocky for the youth involved in the music project. They wanted to work specifically on music and put the rest of treatment on hold. Minnis sent an early message to the youth. If they failed to complete their other treatment assignments, they could not participate in music therapy.

If the youth used profanity or degrading lyrics about women or hate crimes to express themselves, they had to write an essay on why they chose the topic and how it affects them. None of them wanted to do any extra writing so they avoided certain topics. Some of the youth displayed a musical talent that once lay dormant within.

After each musical recording, the youth openly discussed in a small group with Minnis how the music made them feel emotionally. Emotional Expression group evolved into a triumphant event. The youth seemed to prosper and grow daily.

The youth carried the same enthusiasm and positive creativity from the music group over to the Men of Distinction group. During the group, Hawkinson addressed the power of B.E.L.I.E.V.E. to the youth. For many of them it was a concept that did not fit the grid of their programming. Where they came from, there was nothing to believe in. Individuals like Geronimo, Brennen and Sanchez adopted the philosophy right away. They had passion and a drive that separated them from the rest. Most of the others didn't have that drive so it was quite difficult for them to believe in themselves, therefore they didn't accept that they were the best ever living individual evolving very excellently.

Chapter 11
The Coming of Thadius Powers

The non-aggressive youth that hid in the shadows of the more aggressive peers early on during the yellow phase were now starting to expose themselves during the red phase. Thadius Powers was one of those youth. He loved sitting in front of the television with a blank gaze when he wasn't artistically creating.

The youth was undersized for the age of eighteen. He had dark hair and thick box frame glasses. His teeth were slightly bucked and turned inward. His bottom teeth were misaligned. The youth talked fast and often stuttered when he spoke. His ears were pointy and bat shaped. His physical frame was scrawny. His feet were much too big for his body. His clothing always seemed to swallow him up. His peers often expressed that he resembled a combination of Harry Potter, Chucky from the Rug Rats and a bat. Despite all of his physical abnormalities, the youth was one gifted artist.

Thadius Powers was his name, but his peers that were in the Department of Corrections with him knew him as B.A.T., which stood for Bad Ass Thad. Thadius was a terror when he was in corrections. The files read that he spent at least three quarters of his stay in confinement for popping sockets and attempting to start fires. He also climbed rooftops after throwing feces at the guards and youth that picked on him. The list went on and on for Thadius Powers. Eventually he got it together long enough to earn parole.

Since his arrival at the academy, Thadius hadn't said much. During the yellow phase, he spent most of his days and nights observing and downloading the actions of his peers and staff. Thadius also had a crush on Sunflower.

Whenever she needed help on the unit with a task, Thadius was the first in line to volunteer his services. He was always prepared to be of some assistance. Because, Sunflower was kind hearted by nature, Thadius always distorted her kindness into a personal likeness for him and him only.

As the red phase progressed into the shortest month of the year, Thadius became more and more vocal. Because he observed everything, he knew everything. He was starting to hold the other youth accountable for their inappropriate actions. If any of them attempted to intimidate him, he would go straight to the staff. Intimidation in a treatment environment wasn't tolerated. It carried a heavy consequence. Thadius knew this oh too well and he used it to his advantage. The other youth always backed down when he threatened to go to staff about their intimidating threats. None of them wanted to risk violating their parole or probation, especially over Thadius.

Thadius Powers was starting to make a name for himself. He sat back and patiently waited four months to earn a spot at the top of the ranks. His stock had climbed from the last man on the totem pole up towards the top with Geronimo, Brennen and a few of the others. Because, he completed all the required written assignments successfully, Thadius earned a coordinators position. As a coordinator, he allowed the title to go to his head instead of his actions and his heart. He misused the position that was to teach him leadership. Instead, he turned it into a dictatorship for power, not just any power, but Thadius power.

Many of the youth that knew Thadius from corrections struggled to accept his role and identity as a leader. To them, he was still the same neurotic, impulsive, explosive kid that everyone despised. It was only a matter of time before his peers took action against his single party rule.

*   *   *   *   *

One late evening while Hawkinson was sitting in his office preparing the curriculum for the February African American History program, there was a knock at his door. When he looked up, Thadius was standing in the doorway with a twisted bizarre smile.

"What can I do for you youth Powers?"

"It's Thadius and I was wondering if I could hang this drawing up on the wall in the grand room next to Malcolm, Martin and the others for Black History month," he said in a condescending manner. Hawkinson quickly observed the actions the other youth expressed to him about Powers' power and control issues.

"Okay, let's see what you have," Hawkinson said detecting sarcasm. as he waved the youth into the office. Thadius walked into the office cautiously as he studied his surroundings before sitting in the chair in front of the desk.

"Wow, this is cool. If I knew your office was this nice, I would have come to visit you a long time ago Mr. Hawk," he said picking up one of the stress balls on his desk.

"It's Mr. Hawkinson and I'd appreciate it if you wouldn't touch things that don't belong to you," he said mirror imaging the youth's sarcasm.

"Right, sorry Mr. Hawkinson. I don't know what I was thinking," he said realizing his mistake.

"I appreciate the apology. It was much better than the sarcastic attitude you brought into my serene environment."

"Sorry, it's a bad habit that I need to break. I guess I developed it from years of low self-esteem. I learned that in Ms. Sunflower's life skills group," Thadius said as he looked down at the floor and smiled at the thought of Sunflower.

"Youth Powers, when you keep apologizing for the same mistake, it makes you appear unsure of yourself. This is something you're going to have to learn as a future leader," Hawkinson said as he studied the youth's disposition. "Now what is it you want me to hang on the wall?" Powers held up a portrait he designed on an 11 x 17 canvas. Hawkinson accepted the portrait and looked it over before laying it on his desk.

"Did you create this masterpiece?"

"Yes I did," Powers said with a childish smile complimented by a gleam in his eyes.

"Wow, this is remarkably good."

"I know," he said in an overzealous tone as he stared at the portrait. The portrait was of a man/hawk flying over a field of sunflowers with the sunrays of the rising sun illuminating its wings. Thadius sketched every intricate detail to perfection. Hawkinson had witnessed many youth with artistic abilities pass through Lake Apache, but none as gifted as Thadius Powers.

"It's a wonderful creation youth Powers, but if you don't mind me asking, what does this drawing represent?"

"The hawk in the sun symbolizes you. The field of sunflowers symbolizes Ms. Sunflower. You two are my superheros. I've never looked up to anyone the way I look up to you two. It's just a small token of my appreciation."

"Well it's very creative and it's nice to know we have been of some service to you," Hawkinson said looking over the portrait.

"Oh that's not it. I have another one for you," Powers said holding up another portrait. Hawkinson stared at the portrait in disbelief. He and

Sunflower were standing side by side posing with their hands on their hips wearing etheric blue spandex superhero uniforms.

"Youth Powers?"

"Yes Mr. Hawkinson."

"Why does the portrait of me have really big breasts?"

"Those aren't breasts, they're really big chest muscles. Look, Ms. Sunflower has 'em too," Powers said pointing to the portrait.

"Okay, I think it would be best if we kept this one between you and me," Hawkinson said raising an eyebrow. The spandex and "chest muscles" would never go over well with Sunflower.

When Powers' session was over and he was gone from Hawkinson's office, Sunflower entered carrying a stack of files Hawkinson had requested. She sat the files on the chair in front of his desk.

"Wow, nice portrait she said glancing at the art work before turning to leave. Sunflower immediately did a double take when she noticed her face on one of the characters. She walked around to the other side of Hawkinson's desk to gain a closer look.

"Is that supposed to be me?" she asked with her mouth gaped open.

"Ugh, yeah," Hawkinson said trying his best to keep from laughing.

"Why is the chest so enlarged? Better yet, why is your chest more enlarged than mine?" she asked snatching up the portrait and studying it closely. Hawkinson waited patiently for the next question.

"Who created this overexaggerated… piece of work?" she asked.

"Thadius Powers."

"Nasty buzzard," Sunflower mumbled. "This portrait does not leave your office Hawk," she said in a commanding tone as she shoved the portrait back to him before walking away.

*   *   *   *   *

It was the last week of February, the celebration of African American history month. The focus of the group was based on African Americans who had a direct impact on the economic development of the United States and the conscious evolution of civilization. Each youth was to research an individual or group of people and discuss them in detail. It was interesting to Hawkinson how many of the youth arrived to the program prepared and ready to present.

Youth Roosevelt chose to present first. The person he chose to represent was Marcus Garvey. He briefly discussed how Garvey's approach to African American people promoted self-reliance and self-determination. Youth Brennen represented Thurgood Marshall the Supreme Court judge. He did his homework and presented well. Braylon represented Stanley "Tookie" Williams. He discussed how the ex-gang member wrote children's books and had a conscious effect on thousands of American children as well as people around the world.

Several more youth presented. A couple chose Dr. Martin Luther King Jr. Another chose Rosa Parks and talked about the bravery she displayed while not giving up her seat on a public bus in Montgomery, Alabama. One youth from Ohio chose Ted Ginn Sr. the state of Ohio's African American football coach. Ginn is a coach who spends countless days and nights working closely with misguided teens. His "no failure" approach has guided athletes to college and the professional level including Heisman trophy winner Troy Smith of the Baltimore Ravens and Ginn's biological son, Ted Ginn Jr. of the Miami Dolphins.

The last youth to present was Marley Averson, the youth who vowed to return to the Department of Corrections due to the cutting off of his blonde dreadlocks on his first day at Lake Apache. The youth presented his assignment on Malcolm Little aka Malcolm X, the articulate, charismatic speaker. Youth Averson was brilliant in the way he represented Malcolm. He discussed how young Malcolm's dreams were crushed by a teacher who told him he should lower his goal of becoming a teacher or lawyer and stick to being a carpenter or janitor.

Averson discussed how Malcolm dropped out of school and was later incarcerated due to a number of delinquent behaviors. While incarcerated, Malcolm changed his entire thought process and began living life with a purpose. After his release from prison, Malcolm became a symbol for the evolution of political consciousness. Before his assassination in 1965, Malcolm left the entire world with a powerful quote. Youth Averson spoke as if he was Malcolm himself.

"I believe in recognizing every human being as a human being, neither white, black, brown nor red." When he finished speaking, his peers rose to their feet and applauded his stupendous efforts.

The overall program was a success. Hawkinson was amazed at the effort from all the youth. Many of the youth voiced their opinion that the study of African American history should be a yearly curriculum instead of only taking place during the shortest month of the year.

After the program, the youth participated in a soul food feast at the dining hall. The environment appeared hopeful and the food was tasteful. Ms. Maya Sunflower and the staff that prepared the meal gave a history lesson to the youth about soul food. They explained that the person who prepared the meal added the core of their soul and hard work into the feast and that's why it was called soul food. The youth ate like kings at the African American history luncheon.

Later that evening, Averson approached Hawkinson and began a conversation on philosophy and the lifelong quest to inner happiness and peace. Hawkinson found the youth's outlook on life quite interesting. Averson was definitely different from the other youth. He had an old soul. His knowledge base was deep and he had a fondness for the late great Bob Marley. He knew every song the artist ever performed.

Hawkinson, Averson and Geronimo spent the evening enveloped in a very deep conversation about various topics that were far off the radar of most high school students. Others would come around in attempts to join the conversation, but would quickly retreat when they couldn't embrace the heavy topic. Hawkinson appreciated the youths' active minds and inquisitive nature as much as they appreciated his wisdom.

*   *   *   *   *

February was over and in rolled March. It was hard to believe the treatment cycle was already into the sixth month. The youth who were on course to graduate were more than halfway to their destination. Braylon and some of his peers were still struggling to complete the yellow phase. Although they worked diligently to catch up, Hawkinson felt that they would repeat the program as holdovers. He'd seen it too many times with past youth that had fallen that far behind.

Youth Geronimo, Brennen, Franklin, Sanchez, Averson and Powers were breezing right through the red phase. Averson and Geronimo were starting to spend more time with Hawkinson. Both of them had many questions about leadership and life. Hawkinson assisted the youth by answering their questions to the best of his ability. He also challenged them to stop stuffing emotions and to confront their feelings head on. During the yellow phase, Averson never physically acted out. Now that he was peeling back the layers of his emotions on the red phase, the youth grew easily agitated and was starting to grow more aggressive.

One day after school, Minnis challenged Averson on one of the simple rules of the program. Normally the youth would have responded in a jovial manner and would have succeeded following the rule. However, due to stuffing weeks of emotions that he refused to process, the youth snapped at Minnis and kicked a garbage can at him. When Minnis approached the youth to support him, Averson pushed him in the chest. A couple of staff standing nearby quickly approached youth Averson and guided him to the quiet room.

Normally an outburst in such a manner coming from one of the more aggressive youth wouldn't have phased Minnis. However, being that it was youth Averson who never acted out in such a manner, he was highly disappointed. Minnis chose to leave the environment to clear his thoughts. Averson sat in the quiet room thinking about his actions.

*   *   *   *   *

The next morning when Hawkinson arrived on the unit, he read the shift notes from the previous two shifts. He scanned the section that discussed Averson's violent outburst towards Minnis. He shook his head in disappointment. He and the rest of the team of therapeutic counselors took to their post on the milieu.

The youth had finished their morning chores and were preparing for the morning group. Hawkinson spotted Averson in the grand room sitting with the hood of a Lake Apache sweatshirt draped over his head. He looked like the grim reaper. Geronimo was sitting nearby attempting to feed him positive words of encouragement. Averson was unresponsive.

Hawkinson walked close by and observed the youth's state of being. He asked Geronimo to excuse himself. After youth Geronimo removed himself, Hawkinson sat down in the chair next to Averson. He commanded that he remove the hood. When the youth removed his hood and looked at Hawkinson, the pupil of his eyes were coal black. Hawkinson studied the darkness in the youth's eyes before speaking.

"Hiding from what you did is not going to make matters worse or better. It's time you man up and take responsibility for your actions. Did you clean up the mess you made?" Averson looked around to see if any of his peers were watching him before shaking his head no. Hawkinson then asked the remorseful youth if he had plans to apologize to Minnis.

"I want to, but I can't face him," he said looking around at his peers again before a lonely teardrop raced down his cheek and splashed on the floor. Noticing the level of discomfort Averson displayed, Hawkinson stood and told the youth to follow him. Averson stood and followed Hawkinson to his office. The youth sat down before Hawkinson in complete silence. He encouraged the youth to speak out freely about his troubles whenever he was ready.

Chapter 12
March Madness

Averson spoke about the incident that took place with Minnis. He expressed that Minnis wasn't the target of his brewing anger and emotions, he just happened to be in the wrong place at the wrong time. Hawkinson asked the youth what angered him. He didn't respond right away. He sat for a while longer before speaking again.

Averson disclosed that when he was a young child he was diagnosed with seasonal depression that often made him respond in emotionally aggressive outbursts. After the fall, when winter settled in and the sun disappeared behind the thick gray clouds for days at a time, Averson grew extremely depressed. Since arriving to Lake Apache, he kept the condition to himself. He thought that he could control the depression by ignoring it.

Hawkinson asked the youth if he was there instead of Minnis, would he have attacked him in the same manner. Averson said no. He expressed that he chose Minnis because he knew he would accept his behaviors. He admitted to Hawkinson that his expectations and boundaries were much higher than everyone else's and he knew he wouldn't approve of such behavior.

Youth Averson was right. Hawkinson wouldn't have stood for the behaviors. He was a well self-disciplined intellect but there was a side to him the youth knew not to visit. To lash out against him physically went against his soul principle. He had a reputation for challenging the biggest and toughest of the youth who'd come through Lake Apache. He didn't challenge them with brawn, he challenged them with courage, integrity, mental warfare and most importantly, love. Those were the only weapons of mass construction that he used to discipline the youth and help build them up.

Hawkinson was fair. He showed no favoritism to any of the youth. Everyone had to show respect to earn it, from the smallest to the largest, strongest to the weakest and shortest to tallest. It didn't matter the race, culture or ethnicity.

When Averson finished processing his feelings and thoughts to Hawkinson, he returned to the milieu. The youth felt better about himself. The natural hazel color of his eyes returned. A smile softened his face and good vibrations brightened his spirit. He attended group with the rest of his peers and went on to have a positive day. Later during the second shift, he had a long talk with Minnis before apologizing for his ill actions.

The weather for early March soared from below the freezing mark up into the low fifties. Everyone assumed spring had sprung. History has proven that whenever the weather vacillates from one extreme to the next, there is always a change in human behavior. For the youth at Lake Apache it was mostly violent behaviors. Code blue calls over the PA system from the school took place throughout the day.

Every year during the month of March, the youth of Lake Apache seemed to go haywire campus-wide. The month was so chaotic that Hawkinson nicknamed it March Madness. He grew to understand that it wasn't just the youth at the academy, the students at the alternative schools and public schools where he mentored teens carried on the same types of behaviors.

Later that evening the temperature dropped down into the lower thirties. It snowed. Chaotic streaks of lightning lit up the dark sky. Global warming was having a strange and unpredictable effect on the weather as well as some of the youths' behaviors.

During one of the more intense family therapy groups, Joby grew angry as memories from his abusive past surfaced while he was presenting the chronological history of his neglectful family. He exited the group, stormed off the unit and bolted out the side emergency door. Sunflower heard the alarm go off as she exited her office. She grabbed her radio and called a code blue before exiting the building.

Hawkinson dropped what he was doing and grabbed his hooded sweatshirt, radio and flashlight. When he exited the building outdoors, three staff including Sunflower were already out searching the area. Hawkinson caught up to them near the wood line by the parking lot. Snow was falling heavily.

Hawkinson flashed the light on the ground. He kneeled down and studied the fresh footprints of the youth who went into the woods. There were prints next to Joby's. Hawkinson immediately realized the other prints belonged to the coyote. The youth had entered the woods unaware of the dangers that awaited him.

"What's the matter Hawk?" Sunflower asked studying the serious expression on his face.

"He went into the woods where the coyotes dwell," Hawkinson said as he flashed the light into the darkness of the woods. The other two male staff looked at one another strangely and began back stepping when they heard Hawkinson mention the coyote.

"I'm going in," Hawkinson said noticing his two colleagues' reactions.

"Me too," Sunflower said without thinking as she stepped forward. Hawkinson told his two male colleagues to go back and get more help. The two staff retreated after they gladly agreed to go back for assistance.

"You sure you want to come along?" he asked Sunflower who looked as if she was having second thoughts about entering the woods.

"Let's go before I change my mind," she said studying the wood line. Hawkinson reached down and picked up a long thick stick with a sharpened point. He handed it to Sunflower. He told her to stay close. Hawkinson took off through the woods following the footprints. Sunflower was right on his heels. The flashlight illuminated their path. A staff member's voice from another unit came across the airwaves of the radio.

"Unit eight what is your location?"

"We're in the southeast woods across from the main parking lot," Sunflower responded into the radio. The radio frequency began to go haywire. All communication was lost. There was nothing but static. The loss of communication was due to the dense woods. That particular area of woods was a dead zone. No radio communication went in and none came out. The radios and cell phones never worked in "coyote woods" since Hawkinson could remember.

"Oh crap. The radio stopped working Hawk."

"Turn it off. We're in a dead zone. If there are coyote nearby the static will draw them to us."

"And like that big Batman spotlight you're carrying won't. I bet the people in China can see us coming with that thing," she said sarcastically to help ease her anxiety.

"Just turn off the radio Maya," he said refusing to feed into her nervous anxiety. She turned off the radio as requested. Public speaking for many is ranked as the number one fear. Being alone in a wooded area with no means of communication along with coyotes lurking had to rank as number two.

About three hundred yards into the woods, the sounds of a helpless teen yelling out for help followed by the yapping and howling of several coyote rang out. Hawkinson and Sunflower's paces quickened as well as their heartbeats. Hawkinson spotted a pair of glowing eyes in the wood line off to the left from his peripheral. He slowed his pace until he came to a complete halt.

"What's the matter? Why are we stopping?" Sunflower asked studying Hawkinson's slowed movements. He shined the light in the direction where he saw the eyes. The silhouette of a coyote darted past. Sunflower clutched Hawkinson's arm with one hand and tightened her grip on the stick with the other. He followed the large shadow with the light until it disappeared out of sight. Hawkinson reached down and picked up a stick partially covered with snow.

"Let's keep going," he said picking up the pace. The footprints grew fresh as they neared the howling coyote. By the dimension of the coyote prints, Hawkinson could tell the animals were big in size. The March snow continued to fall heavily as if it was Christmas Eve.

Hawkinson and Sunflower began yelling the youth's name. He screamed out their name in return. The two staff quickened their pace even more until they came upon a cluster of interwoven trees surrounded by coyote. The youth was up in the trees looking down at the yipping snarling predators. When the wild animals turned to face the approaching light, Hawkinson and Sunflower halted in their tracks.

With his lighting quick observation skills, Hawkinson quickly took inventory of the number of predators. There were five coyote between thirty-five and forty pounds barking at the youth in the tree. Three coyote weighing between forty and fifty pounds stood guard near a burrow next to an old tree that lay stretched across the earth. Hawkinson flooded the burrow with light. Inside the burrow were two coyote lying down. The coyote by the tree and in the burrow were female and the three guarding the burrow were male.

"It's early March which means breeding season. This kid has no idea what he just stumbled upon," Hawkinson said shaking his head.

"Okay, that would explain why they're so angry, he disturbed their groove," Sunflower said as she caught a glimpse of an approaching figure from the corner of her eye.

"Hawk!" she cried out. A coyote sprung forth from the tree line. Hawkinson immediately blasted the bright light in its eyes. The reddish brown coyote with a black stripe down its back veered off and approached the burrow. The coyote was the largest of them all. It had to weigh between sixty-five and seventy pounds, which was unheard of for a coyote in the state of Illinois.

The massive prowler sniffed near the burrow before peering inside. Once it was satisfied, it began weaving in and out of the other coyote as if it was doing some kind of dance. The large coyote stopped weaving and slowly stepped out in front of the rest. He stared at Hawkinson and Sunflower.

The animal reared its head back and began yapping before letting out a long howl. When it finished, the others in the pack followed suit by rearing their heads back and howling as well. When they finished, all the coyote including the leader raised its leg in unison and began urinating.

"Okay, I didn't sign up for this. What are they doing?"

"Marking their territory," Hawkinson said as he took the opportunity to observe Joby, wedged up in the trees. He was shaking uncontrollably as he stared in amazement down at the pack. Sunflower covered her nose and began gagging as the awful smell of coyote urine penetrated her nostrils. The warm urine from the coyote caused steam to rise up from the ground. The area near the trees became hazy and foggy. The coyote blended in with the haze and temporarily disappeared.

"Hawk, I don't remember reading anything in our job description about us rescuing any youth from a group of pissing coyote. Can we please leave now?" Sunflower asked as she began back stepping preparing to run.

"Don't move. If you run, they will chase you down like prey, and whatever you do, don't look into their eyes. They have been known to attack," Hawkinson said reaching behind him and pulling Sunflower close. For a moment, there was a silent and creepy stillness. Out of the stillness of the haze emerged the lead coyote. He yapped once and slowly began approaching the two staff.

Hawkinson could feel Sunflower's body shuddering against his back. Once again, she attempted to pull away as if she was going to run. Hawkinson reeled her in and held her close.

"What does it want Hawk?" she asked in a stammering whisper.

"I think he's testing us."

"Testing us for what?"

"Trust and loyalty," Hawkinson said with a sheer of confidence. He told Sunflower to ease her fear, because animals could smell and sense it from a great distance. He could slowly feel her body starting to relax, but the fear was still apparent.

"Change your thought atmosphere and think of something positive and relaxing you love to do... like shopping."

"Not funny Hawk," Sunflower said punching him in the back. The coyote stopped within a few feet of the two and began sniffing the air. So that he didn't appear as a threat, Hawkinson lowered the flashlight down towards the ground. He was able to get a good look at the coyote's features from the illuminating light reflecting off the snow.

The snout of the creature was reddish brown like the fur behind its erect ears and the rest of its coat. A blackish stripe traced down the ridge of its back all the way to the tip of its tail. The fur from its neck to its underbelly was a yellowish brown. Its huge paws sank down in the surrounding snow.

The animal was a creation of beauty. It was different from the rest of the light gray and brownish creatures in the pack. The energy radiating from the predator communicated its difference.

Hawkinson raised his gaze from the coyote's feet to its legs on up to its neck and snout until his eyes met the eyes of the wondrous creature. The two stared into one another's eyes where they remained locked as they read one another's intentions. That's when Hawkinson realized the predator before him was the same coyote he first encountered at the edge of the parking lot back during the late fall.

The coyote broke its gaze from the stare down and looked over its shoulder at the youth in the tree. It yapped once. It then returned its attention to Hawkinson and Sunflower before yapping again. Hawkinson slowly nodded his head.

"Hawk, I thought you said not to look them in the eye. What are you two long lost friends?"

"I think he wants to form a treaty, sort of like an agreement."

"I think you've watched one too many episodes of Wild Kingdom." The coyote turned and retreated to the rest of the pack and began yapping. The ten coyote including the two from inside the burrow backed away from the lead coyote and the tree forming a path. The lead coyote stepped aside and looked from Hawkinson and Sunflower to the youth in the tree.

"I think it's giving us permission to go and get him out of the tree," Hawkinson said observing the coyote closely. Hawkinson slowly took a step forward. Sunflower closed her eyes, as she stayed glued to his back. When the coyote didn't respond, Hawkinson took two more steps forward. Still, the coyote didn't move. Hawkinson and Sunflower slowly made their way up to the trees past the two rows of coyote.

Hawkinson turned to face the coyote when they reached the tree, placing Sunflower between him and the tree in case the coyote attacked. He told her to coax the youth down slowly from the tree and for neither one to make any sudden moves. Before she could explain to the youth, he jumped out of the tree and fell into the snow.

Two of the coyote charged the youth snarling and growling. Hawkinson beamed the flashlight in their eyes as he reached down and snatched the youth up by the arm. The lead coyote charged the two snarling coyote yapping. He communicated for them to back down. The two predators wisely backed down.

"Hey, I said no sudden moves," he told the coatless Joby who was so cold that his teeth were chattering loudly.

Hawkinson could feel both Sunflower and the youth trembling from cold and fear as they clung to each side of him. Hawkinson waited patiently for the okay signal from the head coyote. After the leader of the pack finished staring down the two coyote, it looked at Hawkinson in a way as to tell him to move out slowly.

Hawkinson read the coyote's eyes as he began taking baby steps through the ranks of the others. Sunflower and the youth matched his steps the entire way. The lead coyote followed behind them at a distance. One of the more aggressive male coyote stepped forward and began sniffing Sunflower as she walked by.

The lead coyote charged the breeder and yapped loudly. It retreated to the ranks with the others. Hawkinson, Sunflower and the youth continued moving until they were clear of the ranks of the coyote. Hawkinson slowly looked over his shoulder. The leader was gone. The rest of the coyote closed rank and began stalking around sniffing the ground and air.

"Whatever you do, don't look back," Hawkinson said adding emphasis. They quickened their pace along the trail. Every so often, Hawkinson would peer over his shoulder from his peripheral. When they were a nice distance away, he observed two coyote sneaking up behind them.

Hawkinson handed Sunflower the flashlight in exchange for her stick and told her and the youth to run as fast as they could to the entrance. Sunflower looked over her shoulder before accepting the flashlight. When the coyote made eye contact with her, they stopped in their tracks and began snarling.

"Maya! I told you not to look back!" Hawkinson said in an elevated tone. The coyote charged them. "Run!" Hawkinson yelled out. Sunflower and the youth took off running as fast as their aching cold legs would allow. Hawkinson stood his ground and launched the stick. The pointed stick flew like a javelin through the air towards the approaching coyote. The stick descended before connecting with one of the stalking predators. The coyote yelped like a wounded dog as it toppled over.

Hawkinson took off running along the path still carrying the other stick. He followed the light carried by Sunflower up ahead. The other coyote kept coming. It was gaining ground on Hawkinson. He knew it was only a matter of time before the stalker caught up to him.

Hawkinson stopped and turned to face the coyote, raising the stick high into the air. The coyote went into a skid. Hawkinson brought the stick down forcefully aiming for the tip of the prowler's nose. He missed by centimeters as the coyote turned and retreated.

Hawkinson took off running. He could barely see the light up ahead as it grew dim. He knew he must be close due to the voices he heard up ahead. The light carried by Sunflower completely disappeared. Hawkinson kept running hoping to remain on the path.

He slipped and stumbled nearly falling into the bush. The stick flew from his hands and was immediately swallowed up by the darkness. He heard pants from behind in the distance. He kept moving in the direction where he last saw the light. The more he ran the more he heard voices of the people.

Chapter 13

The Misunderstanding of Horus Hawkinson

Forty more yards and Hawkinson was home free. The feeling in his gut told him to turn around. When he turned around, he was met by a set of glowing eyes leaping from the depths of darkness. Hawkinson raised his arms to shield his face as he braced himself for the impact, but the impact never occurred. He heard a thud followed by a yelp and snarling.

Several bright lights appeared from behind Hawkinson. Sunflower had returned with colleagues from their team to aid and rescue him. When he uncovered his face and looked at the ground, the colorful rust colored coyote had the attacking coyote by the throat holding it still.

"Hawk, are you okay?" Sunflower asked slowly approaching. The other staff members stood back as far as possible looking on in amazement at the pretty coat of the lead coyote.

"I'm fine," he said in uttered disbelief as he began back stepping until he joined the ranks of his peers. Hawkinson struggled to process mentally what had just taken place. He kept thinking, *why did the coyote turn on one of its own to spare his life.* The coyote continued to hold one of the members from its pack down by the throat until Hawkinson and his peers were well out of sight.

As the staff from unit eight emerged from the woods with Hawkinson by their side, cheering and applauding from awaiting staff and youth filled the night air. Joby was standing with his peers wrapped in a blanket trembling. Hawkinson approached the youth and placed a hand on his shoulder.

"The next time you decide you want to go on run, how about utilizing that nice track out back," Hawkinson said looking into the startled eyes of the youth.

"O…kay Mr. Hawk…in…son," said the stammering freezing youth. The staff began rounding up the youth to return inside. As everyone was walking away, Hawkinson caught a glimpse of a shadow at the entrance of the woods from his peripheral.

Standing at the entrance just several feet away staring at him with half its body visible was the rust colored coyote. The lighting from the parking lot lamppost gave him a clear view of the coyote. It stared at Hawkinson making direct eye contact. Hawkinson stared in return.

"Aye yo everybody, check it out," one of the youth said in his east coast accent. The rest of the youth and staff stopped and turned to watch what was taking place. The coyote lowered its head to the ground while still watching Hawkinson, and began sniffing the footprints. After it finished its sniffing ritual, it stepped out from the woods fully exposed.

The youth began awing, pointing and commenting on the size of the coyote along with how beautiful its rust colored coat was. The coyote took a step towards everyone. Some of the youth and staff began back stepping preparing themselves to run.

Hawkinson stood his ground. He and the coyote continued to stare one another down. The coyote broke its gaze, lifted its hind leg and urinated at the front entrance of the woods. The many youth lost it as they began laughing and pointing.

"Nasty buzzard," Sunflower said as she shook her head in disgust.

"Hey Joby, he acts like you," the pudgy youth with the east coast accent said laughing it up. After the coyote finished marking its territory, it looked at Hawkinson one more time, before darting away into the woods. Hawkinson smiled to himself before joining the ranks of the youth and staff.

*   *   *   *   *

It was a few weeks later and spring had sprung. The long cold snowy winter had everyone wanting to get outdoors. Mother Nature was doing her thing. The birds sang in the trees causing the trees to bud and bloom. The rabbits hopped around doing the fertility dance with one another in the bushes, and the robins covered the ground to greet the morning sun as they pecked for worms.

The arrival of spring had a great effect on nature just as it had on the creatures that inhabited nature, including the youth. The boys seemed to talk about the girls a lot more than usual and the girls sought attention from the boys. Spring was in the air.

One evening a female rookie staff from another unit decided to walk a small group of girls in front of the male youth dorms. She paraded up and down the sidewalk with girls as if they were back on the block. Their actions immediately had the male youth all wound up.

Sunflower observed what was taking place and informed the male youth they needed to come inside until the girls were gone. Some of the male youth grew angry and began cursing and swearing along with accusing her of being a jealous hater.

Once they were inside, Sunflower called a group and explained to the youth why they had to return to the unit until the females were gone. Hawkinson sat outside of the group observing. A few of the youth continued to harass Sunflower about the situation. After she informed them of their consequences for disrespect, a couple of them immediately stopped. Three of the youth continued to challenge her disrespectfully.

After the group was over, the three youth took off out of the building. A code blue was called. Several staff came out looking for the youth. They were located over by the girls' dorms knocking on the windows attempting to get their attention. The youth were apprehended and returned to unit eight. They were placed on an indoor seventy-two hour restriction.

The consequences the youth earned combined with the lustful attempts towards the females ignited them to act out even more. Later that night two of the three plus Braylon took off again. They returned outside the girls dorms knocking and attempting to peep in the windows. When the staff caught up to the youth, one of them threatened the staff with an iron pipe he picked up along the way.

The local law enforcement were called in to handle the situation. Once the youth realized the seriousness of their actions, two of the three including Braylon surrendered when the police arrived. The out of control youth with the pipe attempted to take a swing at an approaching police officer. He suffered greatly.

The officer sprayed the youth with pepper spray. When the youth continued to fight the officers pulled out their tazer weapons and tazed him a few times before he eventually surrendered. The officers handcuffed the youth and arrested him for attempting to assault an officer with a weapon, obstruction of justice and resisting arrest. The youth was on parole, which meant he was in violation and would not be returning to the academy.

Braylon and the other youth stood back watching helplessly. An evening of fun and games for the youth ended in a night of tragedy. Once again, Braylon found himself in the back of a squad car. Fortunately, he was escorted back to unit instead of the juvenile detention center.

Braylon and the other peer walked onto the unit escorted by the police. The look of disappointment on his peers' faces forced him to bury his chin in his chest.

"I told you he wasn't going to change," he heard one of his peers say to another. The old Braylon would have reacted foolishly towards the peer who made the comment, but instead he humbled himself and entered the quiet room where he chose to remain for the rest of the evening. He sat in the corner of the room and pulled his shirt over his head.

A group was held to give the other youth a chance to address the situation and to vent their frustrations about the chaotic events performed by Braylon and their other peers. Braylon could hear them talking about him from the quiet room. He wanted to burst out of the room and defend himself but he sat quietly taking it all in. From their words and tone, he knew many if not all of them washed their hands of him. He would never admit it to anyone, but Braylon was remorseful for his actions and fearful for his future. He wondered deeply if his probation officer was going to have him violated.

*   *   *   *   *

The next day had come. Everyone gave Braylon the silent treatment. They treated him as if he was a ghost. He had depleted his peers' positive energy. If they continued to put all their energy and emotions into him, they would have none left for themselves. The red phase was the most critical and challenging of all phases. It required internal energy and emotional strength.

Since Braylon's return Geronimo, Brennen and Averson supplied him with the most support. His most recent action was the straw that broke the camel's back. The three most supportive youth on the unit chose to give Braylon space until he decided to better himself. From that point forward, he was the only passenger on his treatment train. Many of his peers began to make small wagers that the youth would not make it to the end of the red phase.

*   *   *   *   *

The change in seasons from winter to spring wasn't only affecting the youth, it was getting to the staff as well. The happy people grew happier and the miserable people grew more miserable. Nature and the change of seasons was the cause of this sudden shift in moods. At times it got so bad that some of the staff members would project their misery in a passive aggressive manner towards others. It just so happened the pendulum of misery was directed at Hawkinson.

The quality of his leadership was attacked along with the relationship he had with many of the youth. Some of the staff complained secretly behind his back that the youth only listened to him, because they feared him. Others said he walked around with a God complex and acted as if he could do no wrong. Hawkinson seemed to be catching the staff's hostile thoughts from every angle. It wasn't the first time he'd been through it and he knew it wasn't the last. He tightned his negative proof vest and continued to free flow.

Hawkinson never played the victim role to any of the situations. He addressed the issues head on during each team meeting and that which he didn't address, he allowed to roll off his back like water off a duck's. He invited those who had issues with him to speak freely so that the conflict could be resolved.

Those such as Minnis, Sunflower and other veterans who worked with Hawkinson long enough, knew that he had the greatest intentions for the youth and enjoyed the working relationship he had with the team. Because of his diehard passion for success, structure and stick-to-it-ive-ness to achieve goals he set for himself he was greatly mis-understood by many.

Hawkinson walked his talk. He searched for the errors and flaws in his character. When he found the errors, he corrected them. He turned his weaknesses into strengths. The strengths he gathered from his weaknesses allowed his sun to shine, even when the skies were gray.

Most of the staff who came aboard with Hawkinson eleven cycles ago were long gone. Many who'd come in a couple of cycles ago were gone as well. He observed so many come and go, but yet and still he remained. He remained like a tree planted by the water, offering his loving deeds for the children that passed through unit eight.

What most of the rookie staff on unit eight and around the academy didn't understand about Hawkinson was that he ventured through the lake of fire and brimstone as a counselor at Lake Apache, better known as hell days. Where the average individual failed or gave up, Hawkinson succeeded and stuck to it. His success came when he learned to listen to the youth without being judgemental of their actions. He showed them fairness and never gave up on them. When they cursed him, threatened to get him fired and carried on like an ogre from the wild, he always gave them space to heal. He did the same with his colleagues when they would carry on with their issues. Hawkinson always gave a person space to deal with their personal issues.

Something he learned while traveling through life was that the only person he could control was himself.

Youth or staff, Hawkinson never allowed himself to delve too deeply into their issues. It was too simple to become a habit. Habits are easy to develop, but not so easy to break. Hawkinson respected everyone. If he unintentionally did something to offend someone he always made room for an apology, but he never apologized for being himself.

Hawkinson's accountability, confidence, consistency and unusual swagger was sometimes misunderstood by the youth and some of his colleagues as someone who could do no wrong. Hawkinson had no favorites when it came to the youth, and he showed no favoritism. The youth respected him greatly for his sense of equality. If the person on the highest phase acted out, Hawkinson held him accountable just as if he was on the lower phase. If a youth had no privileges and was looked upon by everyone as the low man on the totem pole, but made attempts to grow, Hawkinson commended him greatly. There were some youth who required different treatment methods and Hawkinson provided those methods, but never under the umbrella of favoritism.

It was Hawkinson's high expectations, consistency, motivational drive and perseverance for the youth that earned him his reputation and the youths' respect. Even the youth that claimed they didn't like him still showed him respect. When he walked into a room that was extremely noisy, he would stand silently observing the youth without uttering a word. The youth would automatically bring the volume down when they noticed him observing. He would express gratitude with a simple reply of thank you.

Hawkinson didn't earn the respect of the youth and his peers overnight. It was a long process that developed over a period of time. In the early days, his name didn't register on the popularity charts with the youth. He liked it better that way. It made it easier for him to carry out his duties as a professional practitioner. His primary concerns were that the youth were provided a safe structured environment to conduct cognitive behavioral treatment (healing). Anything else was secondary.

*   *   *   *   *

As Hawkinson was walking across the campus to the administration building, he spoke to a couple of his colleagues who were walking in the opposite direction. One of them mumbled a greeting while the other refused to acknowledge him. Their tone and body language told him they were cross.

When he entered the building, he came across another colleague who immediately shifted his eyes to the floor as if he dropped something when he spotted Hawkinson. Hawkinson read the staff's actions in a matter of nanoseconds. He spoke to his colleague. He looked up as if he was surprised to see Hawkinson. He spoke superficially and kept walking.

Hawkinson was too high on the good life to allow their actions to affect him. He chuckled as he thought how immaturely some chose to act. He cautiously approached Sunflower who was standing at copier making copies for her evening group.

"Hey Maya?"

"What's up Hawk?" she asked smiling.

"Nothing much except for the nasty vibes I seem to be attracting.

"What'd you do now?" she asked shaking her head.

"Take your pick," he said still in good spirits.

"You know the history Hawk. It's the same ol' song and dance. Some people just can't do without the drama. You just happen to be in the starring role today. Tomorrow it could be me. Just realize that spring fever is going around. You should consider it a compliment. All great people who do great things become targets sooner or later. Just keep shining like the star that you are. I'll see you later trouble maker," she said humorously before walking away. Hawkinson appreciated Sunflower's ability to always keep it real with him. He treasured her ability to keep it real in an often times superficial environment. Superficial to Hawkinson was equivalent to failing. He didn't comprehend either one.

Hawkinson found what he needed before heading back over to unit eight. The negative energy surrounding the unit was thicker than London fog. He headed straight to his office and closed the door. He pressed the play button on the cd player. The powerful rush of Niagara falls filled the airwaves. Hawkinson escaped to a state of blissful peace as he closed his eyes to meditate to a positive state of being.

*   *   *   *   *

Later while Hawkinson read over the youths' assignments, there was a knock at his door. He carefully approached the door prepared to face whatever negative force that stood on the other side. He cautiously opened it. Standing on the other side of the door with his treatment folder and journal in hand was Braylon. Hawkinson looked over the youth's shoulder then quickly and suspiciously looked to the left and right of him. The youth looked at him strangely.

"You alone?" he asked.

"Yeah Mr. Hawkinson," the youth said smiling at the way Hawkinson was carrying on.

"Who put you up to coming to my office?" he asked with squinted eyes.

"Nobody," the youth laughed as he covered his chipped tooth smile.

"What's the password?"

"Treatment," Braylon said still smiling.

"Alright, come on in," Hawkinson said as he rushed the youth inside and closed the door behind him.

"You're tweeking Mr. Hawkinson. I think you need to lay off the meditation," Braylon said in a full blown laughter. Hawkinson chuckled in his baritone voice as he transformed back to his original self. He could tell Braylon appreciated the theatrics. It was good seeing the youth laugh. Braylon hadn't laughed in a healthy manner since he'd been at the academy.

Hawkinson's ability to express his humorous side made way for Braylon to open up and discuss his current state of being and future plans. For the first time the youth seemed sincere about his plans. The cockiness and arrogance he displayed in the past was gone. Hawkinson could sense a change developing. The youth appeared to be humbled by his last run in with the law and the silent treatment his peers were issuing him.

Chapter 14

Street Life

Braylon opened his journal and discussed what he'd written since his return to Lake Apache just before Thanksgiving. He began with his dysfunctional background. It was the first time in his life that he was giving anyone an up close and personal look at Braylon ShaMar Nicholson.

From day one of his existence, there were no positive male role models involved his upbringing. He grew up with all sisters. His drug addict mother walked out of his life when he was a toddler. His disabled grandmother raised him and his seven sisters on her disability income.

Since he could remember, Braylon roamed the streets looking for some form of male influence. The ones he found introduced him to the street life. They nicknamed him B-Nizzle. He was stealing bikes by the age of seven, and stealing cars driving them to the chop shop by eleven. No one in his family could tell him anything. In his mind he was an adult doing big things.

When the word got out that Braylon was cashing in big on the stolen cars, neighboring street hoods chased and mugged him several times. They took his money and his possessions. The incidents made him bitter, cold and fearful. One day he stopped running and faced his fears. He told Hawkinson that he tucked the insecure eleven year old little boy away deep down inside and became a street warrior.

He selected the biggest and toughest individual out of the group that mugged him to make as an example. He used moves that he learned from football and boxing to defeat his opponent. Braylon showed no mercy. Years of built up anger and frustration went into the battered individual. When the others witnessed his relentless attack, they backed off and ran. Day by day Braylon sought them out one at a time until he received his payback. From that day forth his confidence and swagger grew. He never allowed anyone else to lay hands on him again without receiving their just do.

"What do you have against LaBoy?" Hawkinson asked out of the blue.

"He reminds me of the big lame that used to take my money. The one I chose to make as an example, plus he don't respect women."

"Do you respect women?"

"Yep," Braylon responded without blinking an eye. Hawkinson looked beyond his eyes into the depths of his soul and read the sincerity.

"What makes you respect women?" Hawkinson asked. Braylon expressed that his older sisters took care of him along with his disabled grandmother. One day when he was a very small child, he roamed out of the house into a busy street in pursuit of a basketball. A car came speeding up the street. His oldest sister yanked him back onto the sidewalk out of harm's way. After yelling and cursing him, she hugged him close and kissed him for what seemed like an eternity. He said he would never forget that moment for as long as he lived. It was pure unconditional love that she displayed.

He also talked about a time when he was twelve and stumbled upon a girl from his neighborhood. Braylon said she was being held against her will in an abandoned building by a group of older males. He said they labeled her a bust down girl, because she had low self-esteem and a reputation for allowing just about anyone to sexually have their way with her.

Braylon expressed when he entered the building the wolf pack was corralled around her. She was crying and trying to leave as they verbally degraded her and grabbed all over her as if she was less than nothing.

Not able to stand for what was taking place, Braylon intervened and pushed through the crowd of thirsty lust dwellers. A couple of them attempted to grab him up, but he threw a series of punches drawing blood from a couple of them. There was an older guy there who he once stole cars for. He remembered Braylon and allowed him to leave with the girl. Once he got the girl out of the building, he scolded her and sent her home, but not before ordering her to stay off the streets.

He expressed that a week later the same lust dwellers that he punched from that night set him up. They got word from someone in the streets that Braylon was going to steal a car to make some quick cash. Once he jimmied his way into the car the task force was already there waiting for him. Being that he had already violated his probation a few other times, he was sentenced to do time. Braylon just turned seventeen and had been locked up since he was twelve.

"That's my life and times in the streets," he said closing his journal. Hawkinson applauded the youth accompanied by a smile.

"I commend you for opening up to healing. That took a lot of courage."

"Yeah, it did. I ain't never shared my life story with nobody, not even my oldest sister," the youth said smiling uncomfortably and rubbing his left arm, which is something he did when he was nervous. Hawkinson praised him for standing up against the hoods that jumped him and the lust dwellers that were going to cause harm to the girl in the abandoned building. He told Braylon it took a great deal of courage to do what he did in an environment that was so polluted.

That was Braylon's last assignment before advancing to the red phase. Hawkinson congratulated the youth for advancing into the red phase. The youth lowered his head and let out a long deep sigh. Hawkinson asked Braylon to express what was behind the sigh.

The youth stated that for the first time in his life, he felt a sense of accomplishment. He expressed how good it felt to have opened up. He expressed that failure was the norm where he came from and that success was as foreign as observing a distant galaxy beyond the stars through a telescope. Braylon expressed that for some reason in his own way, he never looked at failure as an option. He said that he was a survivor who was finally on the right path to success.

*   *   *   *   *

It was Hawkinson's morning off from the academy. He entered an alternative school where he mentored three high school students individually. He had to pass through a metal detector before going to the front office to sign in. After signing in, he met with the principal to discuss the progression of the three youths' behaviors. Hawkinson and Principal Ericson shared a great relationship as well as a past. At one point in his career, Hawkinson worked side by side with Ericson at Lake Apache Academy. After discussing the three youth, the two shared laughs and reminisced about their days at Lake Apache together.

It was transitional time when Hawkinson went to meet with the students. The hallways were loud and unruly even with police officers patrolling. The students swore at one another as if bad language was part of the curriculum.

Some of the students made comments to one another about Hawkinson being a probation officer as they observed him walking with the principal while carrying a black leather binder. He led Hawkinson into a classroom where the first student he was to mentor awaited him. The teacher was trying her best to teach through the chaos. The student looked up at the clock, stood and began smiling when he saw Hawkinson. He was happy to escape the verbal madness that swarmed around him as he pulled the hoodie off his head. A girl who had been sleeping lifted her head when she heard the teacher mention Principal Ericson's name. She looked Hawkinson up and down from head to toe.

"Who is you?" the girl with poor grammar asked. Before Hawkinson could respond, Principal Ericson chimed in.

"Chandra what are you supposed to be doing right now?"

"Minding my business and leaving yours alone," she said in a snappy tone as she rolled her eyes and focused her attention back to Hawkinson. While the principal engaged the young lady in conversation, Hawkinson took the time to survey his surroundings. The students were very diverse. Three Hispanic males sat together conversing in their native tongue. A young Caucasian girl popped her gum and spoke in a broken dialect as she held a conversation about the latest music videos with two African American girls. A Caucasian male with glasses sat closest to the door sketching marvel comics. He appeared to be in his own world. Four African American males sat grouped together discussing their street life activities from the night before. Every so often, they would say something rude to the girls, which was their way of flirting. He picked up on all the activity in a matter of milliseconds.

Hawkinson and the student left the classroom. The student gave Hawkinson a pound and thanked him for coming to see him. A police officer patrolling the hallways spoke to the youth in passing. The youth gave him a head nod as they crossed paths. Hawkinson could sense that there was some past tension between the two. Their energies told him so. The student sat at a table near the gymnasium. Hawkinson sat down across from him.

The teen was a bright student with a rough exterior. Missing several days of school due to his constant truancy landed him in the alternative school. Although handsome, he kept a scowl on his face to keep himself safe from the outside world. His personality trait was conscientiousness. He was a thinker. He thought carefully before carrying out any plan. He also had great character which made him very likeable by most of the faculty.

"You look sharp Mr. Hawkinson, but then again you always do," the youth said checking out his mentor's attire. Hawkinson thanked the teen who was always complimenting him. Hawkinson viewed him as a good kid with a good heart who grew up in a rough environment with limited opportunities.

Hawkinson asked the teen how he was doing. He expressed that he'd been struggling in the streets. Although he dropped his flags and no longer participated in gang activities, rival gang members continued to harass him. He applied for a couple of jobs, but no one had given him a call. Home seemed like hell as family members dumped all the responsibilities on him. The possibility of his girlfriend being pregnant was another issue eating away at him from the inside out.

The teen seemed tired and stressed. The usual bright light in his eyes was dim. His braided hair was starting to come undone. Hawkinson could tell the teen had been out all night living the street life. The darkness underneath his eyes was a dead giveaway.

The teen told Hawkinson that he gave him a sense of hope every week that he came to see him. He expressed that it felt good talking to someone who actually cared and didn't want anything in return. Hawkinson allowed the teen to talk and express as much as he needed while he listened with his heart and not with a judging ear.

At the end of the session, Hawkinson always offered suggestions and input that the teen could benefit from. As always, before he returned to class, the teen expressed gratitude to Hawkinson for visiting him. The two embraced as Hawkinson encouraged him to be safe while touring the street life.

*   *   *   *   *

While waiting patiently for the next student to arrive, Hawkinson observed the students in the gymnasium from across the way. The boys and girls cursed like sailors and screamed at each other using obscene language. He secretly wondered who their guardians were.

One young teen who was no older than twelve ran out into the hallway after a basketball. The ball rolled over to Hawkinson. He reached down and picked it up before tossing it to the approaching student.

"Thanks," he said as he caught the ball.

"You're welcome," Hawkinson said as he surveyed the teen in a matter of seconds. His eyes were bright, but fierce. Hawkinson could tell by the look in his eyes he'd seen a lot in his young life. He could also tell he'd already been inducted into the street life. The child looked Hawkinson up and down.

"You a probation officer?" he asked.

"No sir, I provide mentoring services."

"What's that?" he asked tossing the ball up in the air. Hawkinson explained the role of a mentor.

"I need one of those. How can I get me one of those that look like you?" the teen asked studying Hawkinson's shoes. The student Hawkinson was waiting for arrived with a sketchpad and pencils in hand. He sat down next to his mentor. Before Hawkinson could respond to the teen with the ball, a young pudgy girl with a foul mouth appeared at the gym door commanding her classmate in the most derogatory manner to return the ball to the gym. He turned to her and began yelling obscene gestures. The girl gave him the finger as she ducked back into the gym. The child turned to face Hawkinson and the older teen who was staring at him.

"What the hell you looking at punk?" he asked the older teen. "I should throw this ball and hit you in your face," he said raising the ball into the air. The older teen stared him down before flinching hard. The child nearly jumped out of his skin as he stumbled and nearly fell as he ran back into the gym laughing it up. The teacher was waiting at the door and he scolded the boy and the girl before closing the double doors to the gym.

"I can't stand those bad ass little kids. They're going to make me catch another case," he said greeting his mentor with a handshake before opening his sketchpad to do some sketching.

This particular teen was interesting. His personality traits were openness and extraversion. He was very artistic, assertive, attentive, loved music and he was self-sufficient. He was a survivor and according to him, a ladies man. He could never seem to stop talking about how much the ladies adored him and his hair.

He was a somewhat thin kid with handsome features. He wore his hair in fresh neat French braids that draped down his neck to his upper back. He was always well manicured and dressed neatly. He loved watches and always wore the latest sneakers. Like most male teens Hawkinson counseled and mentored, he had hoop dreams. His only downfall was that he couldn't stay in school long enough to stay on anyone's basketball team. The street life had him too. Truancy and fighting is why he was ordered to attend alternative school. The teen told Hawkinson that he was a lover and not a fighter, and all of his fights were out of self-defense. Hawkinson believed the youth. Although he put on a tough act in front of the other students, he didn't appear to have a violent bone in his body.

The teen didn't make much eye contact when his sketch pad was open. He was too busy creating a picture for one of his girls. His art pad was like a part of his flesh. It stayed with him at all times. The teen had a creative eye for art. He could close his eyes for a few seconds, open them and draw anything under the sun. He possessed a natural gift.

Hawkinson had been mentoring the youth for quite some time. He felt open enough to express his current family status as a foster child. He badly wanted to live with his biological mother who'd given up her parental rights when he was much younger. Although he never openly admitted it, Hawkinson could sense that the teen resented his mother for giving him up. His words said he loved her, but his tone and the stress fractures in his voice gave a completely different story. As with most young people who'd been hurt and neglected early on in life, the teen possessed an undercurrent of anger. The source of that anger stemmed from the absence of his mother.

The teen expressed to Hawkinson that he wanted to visit his mother and his sibling in prison, but the foster parents didn't want him to have any connection with them. The teen told Hawkinson he spent most of his days, late evenings and nights in the streets. It was his way of escaping a reality created by someone else. In the streets he could create his own reality. He also expressed that the street life accepted him and didn't judge him for who he was. Hawkinson encouraged him to remain hopeful and to be safe after the session ended.

*   *   *   *   *

The last teen Hawkinson was to meet with was a teen girl that earned her way into the alternative school by fighting, under age drinking, smoking marijuana on school grounds and truancy. She made the male students Hawkinson mentored look like choirboys. Most days she skipped attending the alternative school. When Hawkinson couldn't catch her at school, he'd attempt to visit her at home. If she wasn't home he knew exactly where she was, in the streets. She loved the street life. She was heavily involved with whatever was going on in the streets. That particular day she happened to attend school.

Hawkinson filled out his progress notes from the two previous students as he sat patiently waiting for the teen girl. When she exited the double doors that led from the hallway, he stood and greeted her with a smile and a side hug.

"Look who decided to finally show up to school," he said teasingly.

"I almost didn't. I got a headache. I was out kicking it all night. You look nice as always," she said yawning and stretching as she sat down across from her mentor and lay her head on the table.

"Thank you," he said observing her as he did all the teens. The teen looked as if she had just awakened from a long nap and was ready for another. Her eyes were tight. She wore a wrap around her head to hold her hair in place. Underneath the baby blue cotton sweat suit, the extra long white tee she was wearing extended to her knees. The white designer sneakers on her feet appeared new. She appeared much older than sixteen years of age. The street life had aged her.

"What was going on in the streets that made you want to kick it last night?"

"A party," she answered yawning.

"On a school night? You're supposed to beat the street lights home," he said raising his infamous right eyebrow. The teen began laughing hysterically as she raised her head and looked at Hawkinson in a peculiar manner.

"Mr. Hawk this ain't the olden days when y'all had to be home before the street lights. I party like a rock star seven days a week."

"How are your grades?" he asked smiling and shaking his head.

"They do what they do," she said nonchalantly.

"Are you passing any of your classes?"

"Nope, my teachers don't like me. They're a bunch of haters." Hawkinson listened as the teen blamed everyone for her woes and downfalls. As he expected she took no ownership or responsibilities for her past and current situations. When she finished blaming, she talked about her boyfriend and his baby momma drama. The majority of the discussion was about others instead of her. Every time Hawkinson refocused the session on her, she quickly defocused.

He asked if she came up with the list of short term goals he requested during the last session. She surprisingly pulled the list from her pocket. The first few of her goals seemed superficial and unattainable, but as she continued to run down the list, they developed into more concrete and realistic goals. Hawkinson commended her for completing the task. He encouraged her to begin applying the goals to her everyday life. He also encouraged her to stay in school and out of the streets. The streets had nothing to offer her but trouble.

"You're always looking out for me Mr. Hawk. I always feel better after I talk to you. I'm going to try and stay in school just for you," the teen said as she stood to return to class. Hawkinson encouraged her to stay awake and learn something as he gave her a pound. She waved good-bye as she disappeared through the double doors and down the hallway.

Chapter 15
So Fresh and So Clean

Hawkinson sat in his office listening to a track entitled *Don't Stop Believing*, by the legendary rock group Journey while he looked over the last of the assignments from the yellow phase. All the youth had now advanced to the red phase. Even though the more advanced were soon to reach the blue phase, Hawkinson was pleased to see everyone on the red phase.

Youth Marley Averson was starting to spend more sessions with Hawkinson. He was learning about health and nutrition as well as his own personal spirituality. The youth had a question for every life situation. Hawkinson did his best to answer his questions. Youth Averson was ambitious, inquisitive and persistant. He had all the qualities for success.

One spring evening everyone was outdoors enjoying activities except for Sunflower who was inside spring cleaning her office. She came to the door and asked if a few of the youth would volunteer to help bring some things out to her car. Thadius Powers was the first to come running. The staff standing nearby, halted Powers and chose three other youth who were more responsible and in a higher phase to help Sunflower. That didn't sit too well with Powers as he walked away kicking rocks.

Geronimo, Brennen and Averson were the three to help. Powers watched from a nearby bench as Sunflower smiled at the approaching youth. He quickly distorted the smile as she liked them better than him. When she disappeared indoors with them his mind began to race uncontrollably. He sat on the bench counting the seconds until they returned.

When the door swung open and only two of the youth exited carrying bags, Powers stood to his feet. When he didn't see Averson his heart pounded heavily as he began walking towards the building. Seconds later Averson emerged from the building carrying a box. Sunflower was behind him carrying a couple of boxes. Powers rushed to be by her side as he volunteered to take the boxes off her hands. Unaware of his motives she allowed him to help.

When they reached her car and began loading the boxes into the trunk and back seat, Powers began dictating to his peers how the boxes should be arranged. Sunflower kindly thanked him and told him she was more than capable of handling the situation. Powers persistently continued to dictate. He grew so annoying that Sunflower had to escalate her voice to get his attention. The three youth including Averson stopped what they were doing and zeroed in on the bothersome Powers.

"Dude you need to chill out and listen. You're always trying to take over," Averson said in a calm tone.

"Averson is right Powers, if you're not capable of listening I'm going to have to ask you to return with the others," Sunflower said in a disappointed tone. Powers interpreted Sunflower's constructive criticism as a slap to the face. His distortion was that she was choosing Averson over him. The neurotic angry impulsive self-conscious youth lost it.

"Why are you yelling at me and siding with him? I was only trying to help! You're always taking up for him!" Powers said pointing aggressively in Averson's face. Sunflower looked at the youth unbelievably. To keep from losing his cool, Averson chuckled and looked away. Powers' paranoia allowed him to believe Averson was purposely humiliating him before Sunflower. Powers knew how much Averson loved Bob Marley, so he took it there.

"You keep laughing and I'll kick your fake *I shot the sheriff* Bob Marley wanna be having ass! You fricking suburbanite!"

"What'd you say to me you little retarded troglodyte?" Averson asked dropping the box he was holding as he approached Powers.

"Youth Averson back down," Sunflower said as she stepped between the two.

"You heard me! I called you a fake suburbanite!" Powers said back stepping as he spit past Sunflower at Averson. The spit hit and veered off his shoulder.

"Okay youth Powers, that's enough," Sunflower said dropping the box she was carrying. Before she could intervene, Averson charged and pushed Powers in his chest knocking the squirrelly youth off his feet. He flew backwards and landed on his back. The other two youth stepped up along with Sunflower and grabbed Averson. Powers grew livid. He jumped up from the ground and began swearing and calling Averson every atrocious name he could think of.

The youth was so loud that the other youth and staff including Hawkinson came running to the scene.

When Powers saw Hawkinson, he began walking towards him while pointing at Averson screaming that he wanted to press charges. Hawkinson attempted to calm him down, but the youth was beyond irate. Hawkinson signaled to Sunflower that he was going to remove Powers from the situation while she and the others attempted to calm Averson down.

Hawkinson began to walk away from the crowd luring Powers away with him. The youth was so caught up into being a victim that he didn't realize what the crafty counselor was doing. The more he walked and talked, the further they got away from the crowd. By the time Powers realized he was away from everyone else, he and Hawkinson were standing on the all weather track. The youth looked around wondering how he got to that point.

"I love her Mr. Hawkinson," he said looking out into the vast of nothingness.

"Who do you love youth Powers?" Hawkinson asked with a clueless expression.

"Maya Sunflower," he said looking at Hawkinson with a dumbfounded look as if he should have known. "When she speaks it's as if she writes the song that makes the whole world sing. When I hear her laughter, I want to dance on the ceiling. I'd pay a penny for her thoughts, a nickel for her kiss and a dime if she'd only tell me that she loves me. Mr. Hawkinson, she's once... twice... she's three times a lady. When I first saw her, I thought it was just my imagination... running away with me." Hawkinson stared at the youth in disbelief.

"Youth Powers," Hawkinson said interrupting the youth.

"Yeah Mr. Hawkinson."

"The words that you're using to describe Ms. Sunflower are lyrics from different songs."

"It's the only way I know how to express myself. I'm socially challenged, remember," the very unusual youth said. Hawkinson shook his head as they continued to walk around the track. Powers carried on as he incorporated lyrics to express his feelings for Sunflower. Soon the thought of wanting to press charges against Averson slipped his mind. He had new thoughts and a new idea. His thoughts were to clean up his act in hopes that Sunflower would be more attracted to him. Hawkinson and Powers walked the track until the first evening star appeared above on the infinite blue canvas.

*   *   *   *   *

When Hawkinson and Powers returned to the unit, the other youth were routinely going about the evening. Averson was sitting alone in a corner, journaling with his headphones on. Powers slowly and cautiously approached him. Averson looked up in an uninviting manner. Powers signaled for him to remove his headphones. Averson shook his head no. Powers placed his hands together in the prayer symbol and made a face as if he was pleading. Averson rolled his eyes, sighed deeply and removed the headphones.

"What do you want dude? He asked.

"I want to apologize for spitting on you. I spazzed out for a minute after you called me a retarded troglodyte. I'm not a cave dweller regardless of what you may think of me."

"I called you a troglodyte because of the way you carry yourself and you're not retarded. You're actually one of the smartest cats on this unit, but it don't matter when you carry on the way you do. Look at yourself."

"What's wrong with me?" Powers asked looking himself over.

"First of all you need to get rid of those damn D.O.C. cinema movie screen glasses. Your clothes have more lines and wrinkles than a folded up map. Your hygiene is poor as hell and when things don't go your way you stoop as low as a snakes's belly and spit at people. Dude, those are all the characteristics of an uncivilized troglodyte. If you want respect from others then start by respecting yourself. Here's a little news flash for you, Ms. Sunflower don't like you like that. She don't like none of us like that. I've been down that road before. She's a grown ass lady here to help us, so get that through your thick noggin. Mr. Hawkinson conducts a group once a week on hygiene. You should really take advantage. Apology accepted, now peace out," Averson said as he threw up two fingers before slipping on his headphones and resuming to his music and journaling.

Powers stood for a moment staring at Averson in disbelief before he walked away. He collapsed on a nearby chair and thought long and hard about the advice his peer contributed to him. When it was time for showers, Powers was the first one to take advantage. He washed and scrubbed until staff had to beat on the door and ask him to come out.

Powers exited the restroom with his hair slicked back wearing fresh pajamas that he'd never worn. His peers and staff applauded and whistled. The youth smelled like a fresh bar of soap, deodorant and mouthwash. Youth Powers strolled up the hallway whistling a tune by the group Outkast entitled, *So Fresh and So Clean*. All of his peers, including Averson, joined in and began singing the song. Powers strutted up to Averson with a new attitude.

"Welcome to civilization," Averson said sticking his fist out and giving Powers a pound. Powers pounded Averson's fist as he strutted to his room.

*   *   *   *   *

The next morning when Hawkinson and Sunflower arrived on the unit, Powers was dressed neatly and his hygiene was complete. He even took a little extra time to iron and crease his pants. He wore the new wire frame glasses he received when he first arrived at Lake Apache. Hawkinson and Sunflower both acknowledged Powers by giving him a compliment. The youth's face lit up like candles on a birthday cake. Sunflower then commended Powers for apologizing to Averson the evening before and choosing to take better care of his personal hygiene. When Sunflower checked rooms, Powers' room no longer smelled like corn chips, barnyard animals and halitosis. His clothes were folded neatly and his shoes were aligned under his bed soaking in foot powder. He was at the top of the list for the cleanest room.

"I'm curious to know what sparked the new attitude?" she asked Hawkinson as she looked across the grand room at the youth who was gazing at her through the lenses of his new glasses. He smiled when he noticed her watching him. Hawkinson began chuckling.

"I guess that answers your question."

"Not funny Hawk," she said between her teeth as she gave him a quick nudge with her elbow.

"I bet those new glasses have rose colored lenses," he said chuckling uncontrollably.

"One more comment Hawk and I'm going to secretly sign your name on the overtime list for the female program."

"Okay, I surrender. You won," he said walking away. When Sunflower looked over at Powers, he was still looking in her direction.

"Three second rule youth Powers," Sunflower said from across the room. The youth quickly looked away. The three second rule was a Lake Apache rule created for the youth offenders who had really bad habits of staring at people for intimidation purposes and lust. The sad part is when someone would look at them in return for any significant amount of time, the majority would all but lose it. The rule was to help teach the youth how to engage others without being offensive to that person with their eyes. Powers struggled greatly with that particular issue. He even made some of his peers uncomfortable. When Powers wasn't watching television, he had to be warned about the three second rule from both peers and staff.

*   *   *   *   *

Later that evening after the youth returned from school, Powers asked Hawkinson if he could speak with him privately. Hawkinson looked at the list of names of the youth. Powers was near the bottom. One of his peers at the top of the list who had to work in the dining hall opted to switch with Powers. Hawkinson walked the youth to his office and invited him to have a seat.

"Hey Hawk, can I borrow your shredder, mine is broken?" Sunflower asked from the doorway.

"Sure," he said unplugging the shredder. Powers looked away when he heard Sunflower's voice.

"How are you youth Powers?" she asked taking notice of his behaviors.

"Fine," he said continuing to look in the opposite direction. Hawkinson took notice of the youth's behaviors as well. He then looked at Sunflower. She shrugged her shoulders as she accepted the shredder and rolled it out of the office.

"What's going on?" Hawkinson asked the youth as he sat in silence for a moment before speaking. He shifted in his chair and sighed a few times. Hawkinson waited patiently for the youth to speak.

"I thought my new change would make people recognize me more and give me compliments."

"You were recognized and given compliments by your peers and staff."

"I know but—"

"But what?" Hawkinson asked in a supportive tone.

"But she didn't acknowledge me like I thought she should have."

"She who?"

"You know, Ms. Sunflower. I thought if I changed how I look she would like me more. All she could say this morning was *three second rule youth Powers*," he said mocking her in a feminine tone.

"How'd that make you feel?"

"I felt hurt and embarrassed. I couldn't even look at her anymore after that. A part of me wanted to yell and curse her out, but that would have only made matters worse. I did all of this for her. I hate myself. I'm such a fricking panzee. Maybe I am a troglodyte like Averson said."

"So why should she like you if you hate yourself?"

Powers shrugged his shoulders. Hawkinson explained to Powers that if he wanted people to start liking him he had to start liking himself. He told the youth he had to find a quality about himself, preferably an internal quality and focus on it. Hawkinson told the youth the more he developed that quality the more it would shine. Others would soon notice the quality and compliment him on it, which in return would cause the quality to develop even more and shine even brighter.

Powers sat up on the edge of his chair and zeroed in on Hawkinson's words. He stepped it up and took it to the next level with Powers. He told him he could change his look a thousand more times and he may get a thousand more compliments, but if he never took the time to acknowledge and accept his new look, he would always find himself struggling for the approval of others.

"Mr. Hawkinson what's your secret? Why does everyone seem to like you?"

"Because I like me regardless of what others think about me and I treat others how I want to be treated with the utmost respect. It's all about the power of giving. As a person giveth so shall they receive."

"Sounds kind of lame, but cool at the same time," the youth said as he shook his head in a confused manner.

"You have a lot of growing and maturing to do youth Powers. Until you have love and respect for yourself, you'll never get it from anyone else." The youth wasn't trying to hear what Hawkinson had to say. He had a one track mind and it was set on Sunflower. Hawkinson closed out the session, but not before encouraging Powers to start searching for a quality he possessed within.

Chapter 16
A Walk on the Wild Side

Later that evening before he left, Hawkinson stopped by Sunflower's office to give her a heads up on the relentless creepy crush Thadius Powers had on her. He restrained himself internally to keep from laughing out as he thought about the lyrics Powers sang to describe his feelings for her.

"It's not funny Hawk. I'm getting pretty tired of having to bathe in holy water and rub myself down in garlic before coming to work. Every cycle there's always some kid who thinks he's going to sweep me off my feet and ride me away on some magic carpet." Hawkinson couldn't hold back any longer. He laughed it up, as he thought about the many youth from the past cycles who had it bad for his colleague.

"I can't stand you Hawk," she said starting to chuckle as she crumpled up a piece of paper and threw it at him. The both of them laughed hysterically as they went into their memory museums and drug out all the characters from the past that had a crush on Sunflower.

Something they both discovered early on in their career was that one had to have a sense of humor to get through the mentally and emotionally exhausting days at Lake Apache. There was always something alarming, discusting, sickening and stressful going on. Instead of stressing over situations, Horus and Maya learned to laugh, and laugh they did. Laughter was their source of healing to keep from going insane.

Sunflower chose to meet with Powers to clarify her role as a professional therapeutic youth counselor and his role as a client in a residential treatment facility. Hawkinson would serve as a third party. Hawkinson brought the youth into the office and asked him to have a seat. Powers grinned nervously from ear to ear.

"You have a nice office Ms. Sunflower," he said making small talk.

"Thank you youth Powers," she said observing him closely. Once he was settled, she honed in and began with asking questions. "Youth Powers, do you know why you were called to my office?"

"You wanted to talk to me I guess. I hope it won't take too long. I don't want to miss the cookout."

"Don't worry, you won't miss the cookout. What do you think I want to talk to you about?" she asked. The youth dropped his smile and looked down at the floor as he began fanning his legs back and forth like butterfly wings. Sunflower and Hawkinson both raised an eyebrow simultaneously as they looked at one another. The youth continued to stare at the floor and fan his legs persistently.

"To share how I feel," he said looking up for a brief moment.

"Feel about what?" Sunflower asked putting the sole responsibility on the youth. Powers attempted to spin his way out of the questions, but the routine didn't work with Sunflower, she'd come face to face with some of the best spin doctors that passed through Lake Apache.

Sunflower continued to press the youth with questions until he caved in. Powers told Sunflower everything. He told her how he felt about her. Why he felt the way he felt about her, and when he started feeling that way about her. When the youth finished he sat in silence staring at her.

"Youth Powers the feelings that you have for me aren't mutual. They never have been and they never will be. You are a child in need of therapeutic help. My only responsibility to you and your peers is to assist you on a treatment level and that's it," she said.

"But what about the smiles, the kind words and the way you say hi and you're always asking me personally to help you around the unit," the youth said with a bewildered look.

"Youth Powers I smile and say hi to everyone. If I'm saying hi in any way that makes you to think it's something more behind it then you're wrong. And about the helping around the unit, I've asked everyone to help. You are always the first to volunteer."

"You should have told me no," the youth said in a deranged tone. Hawkinson's alarm went off as he sat up on the edge of his chair. "And what about that laugh, that laugh of yours. It's so... so... so stimulating and erotic!"

"Okay I'm no longer going to entertain this conversation," Sunflower said standing. "This is the way it is and here's how it will remain. You will respect my boundaries which have been set since day one. If you can't respect my boundaries as a professional, a call will be made to your parole officer. I strongly suggest you get more involved with your treatment and less with your fantasies. You also need to write out your cognitive distortions about this situation. When you're done, your responsibility is to get with Mr. Hawkinson in your individual session and go over it thoroughly. The blue recovery phase is coming up really soon. The goal of the treatment team is to keep you on target to graduate. Is that understood?" Sunflower asked in a direct tone. The youth slowly nodded his head as he stared at the floor. Hawkinson was impressed by his colleague's direct approach. He couldn't have handled the situation any better.

"Is there anything you have to say before you're dismissed?" she asked. The youth shook his head from side to side in a childlike manner. "Okay, return to the milieu." The youth slowly stood and trudged to the door with his head down. Hawkinson walked him back out into the milieu, but not before turning and giving Sunflower a thumbs up. After walking Powers out, Hawkinson returned to Sunflower's office.

"Well, if I may say so I think you handled that very therapeutically."

"I don't know, this is starting to get a little old Hawk. If I had a penny for every time I gave that speech to a youth, I could buy that nice piece of land back home in Arizona that I've been wanting," Sunflower said as she sighed deeply from mental fatigue.

"It is what it is. Don't let it eat away at you. I'm going to tell Minnis and the second shift to keep a close eye on Powers. He may have an aftershock. I'll see you tomorrow."

"See ya Hawk. Hey, thanks again for the support."

"That's what team members are for," he said before exiting the office. As Hawkinson entered the milieu, he heard Minnis attempting to restore order to a chaotic environment.

Hawkinson approached one of his colleagues and asked what was going on. She gave the report that Powers had gotten into a verbal dispute with a peer over a hotdog. The situation then turned physical. When Powers heard that there was only one hot dog left before the next batch would be ready, he attempted to take one of his peer's food and a fight broke out. Hawkinson asked where Powers was located. The staff pointed to the exit door that led outside. Hawkinson approached the door and heard Powers repeatedly screaming that he was going to take a walk on the wild side. Sunflower came running when she heard the ear piercing screams.

Hawkinson and Sunflower stepped outdoors. A trail of overturned plastic chairs and blood drippings illuminated by the bright sun was the first thing the two counselors observed. The food on the grill was left unattended. The mini boom box sitting on a picnic table surrounded by plates full of food was playing music, but the table was ghostly empty. It was as if the entire area was deserted. Hawkinson and Sunflower followed the bizarre animal like noises coming from around the corner. A staff and a few youth were huddled together staring at something in a corner of the building.

When Hawkinson and Sunflower approached the scene, Powers was squatting down in a shaded corner of the building gripping a few hotdogs he'd snatched off the grill. He was holding the piping hot food with two hands eating away at it savagely, while burning his mouth from time to time. Blood trickled down from his nose onto his lips. Charcoal smudged his hands and face. His ears stretched back and his teeth showed as he snarled intensely. He looked like something from the show, *Ripley's Believe It or Not.*

Sitting on the ground between his legs was a stuffed polar bear he'd stolen from a peer's room before making his way outdoors. The youth made prehistoric grunting noises while he ate. Hawkinson asked his colleague to remove the other youth from the scene and take them back around the corner to the cookout and to send more male staff to the scene. Powers' records reported that he didn't do well with females when he morphed into this particular state of being.

"Mr. Hawkinson, I just want to warn you that he's been screaming that he's about to take a walk on the wild side," a youth who once shared a cell with Powers in corrections said.

"What's the wild side?" Hawkinson asked.

"Excuse my language, but it's when he goes ape shit, literally," the youth said before scurrying away with his other peers. Sunflower looked at Hawkinson in a very concerned manner as he began cautiously approaching the transformed youth. Powers slowly began to rise out of his stance with every step Hawkinson took towards him. Taking notice of the youth's movement, Hawkinson stopped. The youth slowly went back to his crouching position as he glared evilly at Sunflower.

"Youth Powers how about coming out of the corner so you can eat your food at the table and I can get you some buns and condiments to go along with your hotdogs. I'll even get you a napkin to wipe off your hands and a soda to wash the food down."

"Nope, I don't need any stinky buns and soda. I'm gonna stay right here and finish my food," he grunted before belching loudly. The belch reverberated from the corner of the building causing a loud echo.

"Alrighty," Sunflower said as she looked away in a disgusted manner.

"Hey hawk head, you and that stinky snot weed by your side that everyone calls a sunflower ever take a walk on the wild side?" the youth asked belching again.

"How about coming out of the corner and telling me all about the wild side?"

"Nope, I can tell you from right here, and stop trying to read my thoughts hawk face. I know how you operate," he said smacking loudly. The youth finished off the last of the hotdogs as he licked his charcoal stained fingers. "There are no rules on the wild side. All spoils are fair game on the wild side," he said looking at Sunflower with a sickening lustful eye. She squinted and folded her arms displaying no fear. Realizing she wasn't the least bit intimidated, he refocused his attention to Hawkinson.

"You know what I discovered since rejoining the wild side!" the youth said yelling madly. "I discovered you're not a hawk, you're a pigeon! Not just any pigeon, but one of those sneaky shitty city pigeons who likes to crap all over people's dreams! You crapped on my dreams pigeon man! You know what else I discovered since returning to the wild side? There are no sunflowers on the wild side, there are only stinky snot weeds!" he said pointing aggressively at Sunflower.

"I'm the ruler of the wild side and whatever I say goes you fake ass superheroes. There's even dark magic on the wild side. You ever seen a polar bear turn into a grizzly bear right before yo very eyes?" he asked picking up the helpless stuffed animal by the neck. Sunflower raised an eyebrow as she and Hawkinson both began inching themselves away from the shadowy shaded area and more into the sunlight.

"I got a new name for the dynamic duo… Pigeon Boy and Snot Weed Girl. I want my portrait back. I need to do some reconfiguring," the mentally disturbed youth said as he unbuttoned the front of his pants and stuffed the grizzly bear down the back of his pants as he began grunting and making faces.

"Hawk, I think I'm going to go now," Sunflower said back stepping even more.

"Maya, there is no I in team. We're in this thing together," Hawkinson said closely monitoring the youth. When he looked over his shoulder, Sunflower was gone. She'd departed without so much as giving it a second thought. Minnis and two other male counselors approached Hawkinson and stood behind him. They were all wearing safety gloves. Minnis handed Hawkinson a pair of the gloves. He slipped them on and stood back patiently awaiting the youth's next move. The purpose of wearing the gloves was for their protection against any of the youth's bodily fluids in case of a physical restraint.

"Hey Dennis the Menace, you and the other two stooges are just in time for the *Take a Walk on the Wild Side* magic show," the youth said to Minnis extracting the stuffed animal from the rear of his pants. Just as he said, the youth had turned the polar bear into a grizzly bear. The stuffed animal was covered in feces. Powers hurled the stuffed animal at

Hawkinson and the other male staff. Simultaneously they all stepped aside as the stuffed animal whizzed by their heads. The smell was horrendous. Hawkinson's eyes watered.

"The party has just begun you Lake Apache egg heads," Powers said as he focused on the music playing from the boom box around the corner. A song entitled *Walk It Out,* by D.J. UNK was playing. The youth slowly stood from his stance and buttoned his pants.

"That's my shit!" he said as he threw a hand above his head striking a John Travolta pose from the *Saturday Night Fever* movie. He came out of the pose in slow motion as he began his version of the walk out dance routine. He shuffled his feet, swayed to the left, paused and bent at the knees. The youth flung his arms out and threw his head back before snapping his fingers. He repeated the process by swaying to the right. Hawkinson, Minnis and the other staff all looked at one another in complete amazement. Powers had not an ounce of rhythm, which didn't seem to phase him. He danced his routine and walked it out until the song ended. When it was over he began yelling encore over and over at the top of his lungs as he dropped to his knees with his arms stretched out wide.

"Are you not entertained?" he screamed out.

"Youth Powers how about walking it out inside with us, so you can clean yourself up?" Hawkinson asked.

"Stop talking to me chicken hawk pigeon boy! You sold me out to stinky snot weed girl. How could you betray me?" the youth asked in a neurotic dramatic fashion. "From now on I am known to you as Sir Thadius Nicodemus Powers of the wild side. And do you know what time it is?" he asked rising to his feet with a sinister type smile.

"What time is it Sir Thadius Nicodemus Powers?" Minnis asked feeding into the youth's theatrics.

"It's time... to go to the wild," the youth said as he took off running towards the woods. Minnis and one of the other staff took off after Powers. Hawkinson always thought in angles, so he and another staff took off at an angle to head the youth off. Powers realized he wasn't going to reach the woods before Hawkinson, so he detoured and ran in the opposite direction.

Powers spotted an old television antenna on the side of one of the buildings. He scaled the antenna with ease as he climbed onto the roof of the building. The staff approached and asked the youth to come down. Powers refused as he taunted the staff by yelling out obscene gestures. Each time a staff attempted to approach the antenna, Powers ripped off a shingle and flung it down at them as if it was a Frisbee.

Hawkinson instructed the staff to back off. Powers continued to yell out obscene gestures and curse the staff as he put on an award winning performance. Hawkinson decided to take his audience away. He asked Minnis and the others to return to the cook-out, but to keep their radios on and to be on alert in case their assistance was needed.

When they walked away Powers yelled for them to come back. Once they were gone he focused his negative energy towards Hawkinson. The counselor pulled out a small book from his back pocket and began reading. Hawkinson was really good at planned ignoring. He possessed the strength to invert his attention and block out whatever was going on around him. Powers knew this oh too well, but he refused to be ignored. He continued to scream obscene gestures at the top of his lungs toward Hawkinson, but the unruffled Hawkinson continued to read as if Powers wasn't there.

"Hey you muscle bound ninja turtle! Yeah I'm talking to you mister the sun is always shining. Mister hawk in the sun. You're not a hawk in the sun, you're a pigeon in the coop. Hey pigeon head! Do you wanna see my moon make your sun disappear?" the mentally disturbed youth asked while dropping his pants and mooning Hawkinson. Yet, the humble servant continued to read his book and ignore the troubled youth.

When Powers realized the phase of his full moon couldn't stop Hawkinson's sun from shining, he pulled up his pants and sat on the roof top staring down. Periodically, Hawkinson observed the youth closely from his peripheral. The youth laid back and rested his hands behind his head as he stared up at the clear blue sky. Minnis returned to check on his colleague. Hawkinson confirmed that the situation was under control. Minnis returned to the cookout.

Powers sat up and stared down at Hawkinson who was still reading. The youth stood and walked over to the antenna. Hawkinson watched him climb down the antenna from his peripheral and slowly make his way over towards him.

"Excuse me Mr. Hawkinson sir," the youth said in a humble tone.

"Yes youth Powers," he said closing the book and reading his eyes for any cunningness.

"I'm ready to go get cleaned up," he said shamefully as he looked at the ground. Hawkinson asked the youth what was his plan after he cleaned up. Powers paused before speaking as he kicked at the grass and dirt beneath his feet. He expressed that he was going to clean up the mess he made and find a way to apologize to his peers and replace the stuffed animal that he transformed into a grizzly bear. Then he expressed that he would apologize to all the staff for disrupting the cookout.

"That sounds like a good plan youth Powers. I'm ready to proceed when you are," Hawkinson said holding his hand out for the youth to walk ahead of him. The youth took a few steps, stopped and turned to face the modest disciplinarian. He told the counselor he would mostly like to apologize to him and Sunflower for degrading them and betraying their support. Hawkinson explained to the youth that he betrayed himself and he shouldn't apologize unless it was from his heart and not from guilt. The disturbed youth listened closely as Hawkinson continued to educate and counsel him.

Chapter 17

I Believe I Can Fly

(The Blue Phase)

It was May and the youth were now in the third and final phase of the program. The blue phase focused on the recovery process of treatment. Any time treatment is applied, there has to be a recovery process, when one returns to a healthy, stable condition. For many of the youth, the blue phase was going to be their most trying time.

It was a late evening when Hawkinson sat before a group of seven youth to conduct a relaxing meditation group. The purpose of the group was to teach the youth deep breathing, total relaxation, focus and concentration, which would help them release anger, stress, strife and worry. Since the youth were giving up the harmful ways of living, Hawkinson's responsibility was to replace it with something healthy and helpful.

The seven youth sat in a horseshoe shaped format. Another staff acting as co-facilitator sat in the back of the group observing. The lighting in the room was dim and perfect for the experience. Two etheric blue lamps glowed mysteriously. Playing faintly in the background on the stereo was a Native American flute and wooden chimes. The music was to help the youth settle into a relaxed state of mind. Hawkinson explained to the youth that if any felt like journaling instead of closing their eyes to relax, it would be their choice. Since many of the youth carried deep seeded trust issues, it was paramount that he offered them that option.

Surprisingly, all the youth closed their eyes. The music accompanied by the deep soothing calmness of Hawkinson's voice guided them to an inner place of peace. Some of the youth struggled to relax as their bodies wiggled and wormed around in the chairs. The movement was contributed to nervousness, anxiety and fear of the unknown.

In the beginning stages of the group, Hawkinson escorted the youth to a special place in their imaginations. The place was an open grass field with a large waterfall in the distance. The sun was shining brightly. A large limestone rock aligned with alabaster in the shape of a throne sat in the middle of the field. Hawkinson guided the youth to sit upon the rock, but not before looking down and feeling the soft warm grass underneath their feet. This procedure was to help the youth get in touch with and unlock their inner feelings

The once uncomfortable youth were now calm all except one. The one was Braylon. He opened his eyes and observed everyone else relaxing. He looked at Hawkinson who had his eyes partially closed, but was still aware of his surroundings. He then looked back at a staff who had her eyes closed. Braylon's eyes darted nervously towards the stereo playing the music. He then looked at the dim blue lighting before standing and going over and leaning up against the wall. Hawkinson allowed the youth to stand as long as he wasn't disturbing the others.

Once the youth were sitting on the rock in their imaginations, Hawkinson asked them to allow the warmth of the sun to absorb them. He watched through his partially closed eyelids as the youth formed smiles upon their faces. The smiles cracked and broke away the frowns from years of anger, disappointment, horror and trauma. When Braylon saw many of the youth smiling with their eyes closed, he grew a little more comfortable as he went back his chair and sat. He closed his eyes to relax.

In the same low key, but deepened voice, Hawkinson asked the youth to imagine wings growing from their backs as they sat upon the throne of healing. He then asked them to gently flap their wings and allow the air beneath to lift them from the throne. Once they were suspended in mid air with the throne beneath them, Hawkinson encouraged the youth to focus their keen vision on the waterfall ahead in the distance.

Hawkinson focused on Braylon who was now breathing deeply and slowly starting to relax. His once hard cold structured face of anger from years of heartache and pain was now warming and taking on a youthful appearance. The humble counselor instructed the youth to fly towards the waterfall. Once they reached the waterfall, he encouraged them to swoop down and discover whatever was down below in the valley.

*   *   *   *   *

The meditation period lasted for about thirty minutes. Hawkinson began a countdown from ten to zero when it was time to bring the youth back from their place of peace. Most struggled to return from a place so serene, but when they did they returned feeling weightless. Their eyes appeared clearer, faces smoother and their auras didn't appear as murky as before the meditation.

After the youth sat in silence recovering from the spiritual encounter, Hawkinson asked if any of them would like to share their experience. One by one they all raised their hands high into the air until all were raised. In past cycles, very few youth shared about their experience during the first session. This group was special. They took a strong interest in learning how to relax and heal from within.

*   *   *   *   *

Later while Hawkinson was in his office completing the notes from the previous group, Averson arrived for his session. The counselor waved him in. The youth sat before Hawkinson smiling the entire time.

"You okay youth Averson?" he asked putting his notes aside.

"I'm cool Mr. Hawkinson, just feeling the effects of that meditation group. That was real nice the way you guided us to the throne with the wings. I felt like I was really flying. What do you call that technique?"

"CVI, creative visual imagery. Ancient warriors from the past used the technique to heal themselves from any form of sickness and to prepare themselves for battle. The mind is a very powerful tool. As well as it works *for* you, it can work against you. It all depends upon your degree of thinking and creative visualization."

"You're a deep dude Mr. Hawkinson. I ain't never met anybody like you in my life. I used to smoke and get high on the regular. No high I ever had compared to the high I had today. And it was legal," youth Averson said smiling as he rubbed the naturally curly hairs on his head. Hawkinson chuckled at the youth and his refreshed appearance. Since hydrating himself by drinking more water and changing his diet as Hawkinson encouraged him to do, the youth was starting to lose weight and grow more health conscious. He was looking extremely healthy. Between youth Geronimo and Averson, the two inquisitive youth were keeping Hawkinson on his toes with the many questions.

Averson expressed to Hawkinson that he wanted to discuss his experience during the meditation group. Hawkinson allowed the youth to proceed. Averson, like the majority of his peers, never had a relationship with his parents. They walked out on him early on in life. After flying towards the waterfall in his imagination during the meditation group, Averson discovered himself when he was a small child. He was with his parents at a park. The both of them took turns pushing him on the swing set. He was happy. It was the happiest day of his life. Afterwards each parent held one of his hands as they swung him in the air. His mother laughed joyfully while his father encouraged him to swing higher. The youth went on talking about his created visual experience.

When youth Averson finished, he was in tears as he sat in silence. Hawkinson encouraged the youth to embrace the experience in his imagination and to hold onto it. He told him the tears were appropriate and he should allow them to flow for as long as they needed to. The youth raised his hood and pulled it over his head. He continued to sit in silence as he cried a river. When the session was over, he quietly gathered his things. The tears dried up and a smile returned to his face as he thanked his mentor for the session.

"Thanks for teaching me how to get high and fly without using drugs Mr. Hawkinson. I now have a new coping skill that I plan to use quite often."

"You're quite welcome," Hawkinson said as he stood and gave the youth a firm handshake and a fatherly embrace. When Averson was gone, Sunflower appeared at the door. She noticed Hawkinson staring off in deep thought.

"Hey, you okay?" she asked bringing him back to the moment.

"Yeah I'm fine. I was just thinking about some things," Hawkinson said as he rubbed the center of his forehead continuously."

"Powerful session, huh?" she asked.

"Yeah, I haven't had one like that in awhile. It kind of snuck up on me."

"You need to talk?"

"Nah, I'm fine."

"Are you hungry? I'm going out to get something to eat."

"Now that, I can say yes to," Hawkinson said leaving the building to get something to eat, but most importantly some fresh air. Sometimes counseling sessions could be very overwhelming.

*　　*　　*　　*　　*

When Hawkinson returned, he had one session left for the evening. Youth Geronimo Coltrane sat before him in his office with a notepad and pen. The youth was writing down the steps to learning how to relax and meditate on his own. He and Averson were like the Doublemint twins. The both of them enjoyed their one on one time with Hawkinson. They asked a million and one questions, but most importantly, they had a desire to learn.

After Hawkinson gave Geronimo the steps, he asked him what he hoped the meditation process would bring. Geronimo expressed he wanted to gain inner peace with the hopes of being able to control his anger, anxieties and heavily distorted thinking patterns. Hawkinson asked the youth what his plans were once he graduated from Lake Apache. Geronimo sighed deeply and looked down at the floor.

"I don't know," he said returning his gaze to Hawkinson.

"A man who fails to plan... plans to fail," Hawkinson said looking deep into the youth's eyes. "Not having any goals or plans is what landed you here in the first place. Idle time is the enemy's playground. Do you know who the enemy is youth Geronimo?"

"Those who try to pull me into negative situations," he answered.

"Yes, but there's an even greater enemy," he said smiling. The youth looked at Hawkinson with a very peculiar eye. "You and your negative self talk during idle time is the greatest enemy of them all. No one can make you do anything without your approval. When you're sitting around bored and doing nothing is when you're preparing to invite the enemy into your life." Hawkinson introduced the youth to positive affirmations.

He told him that affirmations are affirming statements which lead the conscious and subconscious to accept that which it believes. If a person mentally repeats negative things about themselves, knowingly or unknowingly, they begin to store these beliefs deep within their system. It's the same for storing positive statements. Eventually your system begins to believe what you have fed it. The youth leaned his head to one side as Hawkinson shared the information with him. The head leaning was a sign that the session was getting heavy.

"Who do you blame for being in your current situation?" Hawkinson asked. The youth thought about the question before responding. He then spoke, blaming his drug addicted mother, his hateful foster father who used to beat him for any little thing and his older brother who blamed him for everything and set him up for more beatings from the foster father.

Hawkinson explained to the youth that it was okay to be upset or disappointed with his family, but if he continued to blame them he would be robbing himself of joy and happiness. Once he stopped blaming, only then would he start to grow. Maybe one day he would even learn to forgive. Hawkinson discussed how not to live life as a victim. He told him that if he put himself in the role of a victim, others would treat him as one.

"What do you mean by victim?" the youth asked. Hawkinson explained that a victim is someone who always blames others for their mishaps or unfortunate events.

"Metaphorically speaking, victims drive a little raggedy victim mobile, which is their constant complaining and poor me attitude. They drive their victim mobile or poor attitude down sob story highway. They park their victim mobile in front of their victim hut in victimville which is their state of mind. The world is full of victims driving victim mobiles down victim highways to their victim huts in victimville."

The youth chuckled at Hawkinson's analogy, but thought about it heavily.

"I've never seen you act like a victim Mr. Hawkinson. Why don't you ever complain or get upset about anything?"

"It's easier to not complain and channel that energy into solving whatever issues I have at the time," Hawkinson said smiling.

"You make it sound so easy."

"It is once you practice the habit." The youth sat quietly thinking. Hawkinson could see his wheels turning. He asked the counselor if he had any enemies. When Hawkinson confirmed that he does, the youth's eyes lit up like coals in a fire. He sat up on the edge of his seat eagerly waiting for the response as he pressed his pen upon the paper to take notes. Hawkinson expressed that goodness is his enemy and greatness is his ally. Mediocrity is his enemy and perfection was his ally. Laziness is his enemy and ambition was his ally. Quitting and giving up are his enemies and being a successful champion was his ally. The youth wrote everything down as he smiled.

"You have a lot of enemies Mr. Hawkinson."

"Yes I do youth Geronimo, but I have just as many allies if not more. Without the enemies I wouldn't have any allies."

"You're one unusual cat Mr. Hawkinson, but I like your style," the youth said as he reached across the desk and shook his mentor's hand. Hawkinson commended the youth for having a great session and encouraged him to no longer place himself in the role of a victim.

*   *   *   *   *

A few days went by. Hawkinson was approached by youth LaBoy who had been extremely low key for the past several weeks. Hawkinson made the youth aware that his ban to all female staff was over. Hawkinson looked the youth square in the eyes and asked him what he planned on doing about restitution. Youth LaBoy expressed that he wanted to formally apologize to Sunflower and the other female staff for his immature and disrespectful behaviors.

When his session was over with Hawkinson, LaBoy approached Sunflower and the other female staff. His heart beating so heavily, it could be heard pounding like a war drum from miles away. The youth was so nervous he didn't know how or where to begin. LaBoy had never actually had a real open, down to earth conversation with a woman, especially women of their caliber. He stumbled over his words as he attempted to right his wrongs. None of the women bailed him out as they patiently waited for him to finish. When he finished, Sunflower and the other staff gave input before accepting his apology. The youth thanked them all before walking away. Hawkinson was standing across the room observing as he always did. He smiled and gave the youth a thumbs up for righting his wrongs.

Chapter 18
Trying Times

Hawkinson sat in his office peering across his desk. Sitting on the other side of the desk was Braylon Nicholson, who was gritting his teeth as the muscles in his jaws moved up and down. The youth had just gotten into a verbal dispute with a peer that nearly turned physical. Hawkinson had given him one of the stress balls on his desk. The youth squeezed the ball until the muscles in his jaw began to relax.

"You ready to talk about it?"

"Ain't nothing to talk about. I was about to give dude a pumpkin head," the youth said.

"What would that have solved?"

"He would have stopped running his mouth."

"Maybe, maybe not. Are you going to give everyone who disagrees with you a pumpkin head?"

"Come on Mr. Hawkinson, why are you trying to make me out to be a tough Tony?"

"I'm not. I'm only responding to the comment you made. You ever thought about taking a break from the aggression and violence and shutting yourself out to self-hate and opening yourself up to self-love? You lack love where you need it the most youth Braylon, in your heart."

"Why are you always talking about love? Love is weak."

"Maybe that's because you never experienced it."

"Have you experienced it?"

"Everyday," Hawkinson said smiling. I always start by loving me, because it allows me to love others. Love is a positive winning attitude that I have about myself, which transfers over to others." The youth took time to think about the response before asking his next question.

"Why are you always sitting in the sun… is the sun love?" the youth asked suspiciously.

"The sun gives us life so that would make the sun love." The youth sat quietly thinking about Hawkinson's response before he chose to debate it. The two of them went round and round and back and forth as they debated. Hawkinson liked that quality about Braylon. The youth wasn't simple, he was a thinker, which reminded Hawkinson of himself when he was a youth.

Braylon switched the focus of the session to the meditation group. He shared that it was the weirdest event he had ever experienced. Hawkinson told the youth that when he was meditating, his entire face transformed from being tense and angry to relaxed and peaceful. Hawkinson asked if he was afraid of peace. The youth sat quietly thinking about the question.

He admitted that he'd never experienced peace in his life. Everything since he could remember was chaotic. He discussed in detail what took place during the creative visual experience while meditating. Braylon explained that when he reached the waterfall and swooped down in the valley as instructed, it was pitch black. All light disappeared. His wings felt heavier. As he continued to fly through the darkness, a flash of light lit up the valley below. Tombstones aligned the valley floor. One particular tombstone lit up in red burning flames. The youth expressed that his name, date of birth and R.I.P. was etched in the tombstone and while flying over the gravesite, his family was huddled around the grave dressed in black while mourning.

"What has been your biggest fear since you can remember youth Braylon?"

"Death," the youth said without hesitating. "What I fear the most is dying before getting a chance to live my dream," he said as his voice cracked. He raised his hand to shield his eyes. A lonely tear trickled down his cheek but quickly disappeared. Hawkinson gave him some time before he proceeded with the next question.

"Do you have a death wish?" he asked the youth.

"Sometimes. Sometimes I wish I was dead so I wouldn't have to deal with the pain."

"What pain?"

"The pain from the things I saw and experienced while growing up. I was supposed to be dead a long time ago," the youth said as he dug his index finger into the side of his head as if he was trying to bore out the thoughts. Hawkinson expressed that he would provide him with created visual techniques to help delete the deep mental impressions that preoccupy his thoughts.

*   *   *   *   *

Like staff at similar institutions, Lake Apache's staff usually experienced burn out by the month of May. Everyone, including administrators, counselors and teachers experienced the burn out syndrome. Studies showed that the burn out syndrome occurred more during the month of May due to it being so close to the end of the school year and the weather starting to warm up. Educators and students both would much rather be outdoors enjoying the weather.

With just two months to go, the burn out syndrome was starting to take over the counselors and youth at Lake Apache. People were snappy towards one another. Hawkinson watched the burn out syndrome work its way through unit eight and the rest of Lake Apache Academy like an airborne virus. The number of physical restraints increased. The number of youth attempting to run away skyrocketed and the number of staff call-offs soared.

Every cycle was the same old song and dance. Hawkinson watched as the epidemic affected most around him. He kept himself immune to the outbreak by upping his self-care tactics. He meditated more to slow and ease the disruptive thoughts. He worked out and ran more to take off the edge. It was trying times and those times were getting the best of everyone. Only the strong survived at Lake Apache and the weak perished along the wayside.

*   *   *   *   *

Hawkinson sat in his office working diligently on an individualized meditative treatment plan for Braylon, while listening to a track by Eric Clapton entitled *Change the World*. Sunflower knocked once as she entered his office and plopped down on a chair. She sighed deeply.

"You okay?" he asked looking up from the report.

"Don't mind me. I just needed to be in a serene environment. Everyone seems to be suffering from the burnout virus. The energy out there is so negative," Sunflower said massaging her ear lobes with her fingertips. Hawkinson observed her actions from his peripheral.

"What are you doing?" he asked chuckling.

"I'm trying that woo-sa thing that you're always doing," she said continuously squeezing her ear lobes. "Woo-saaaa...woo-sa-laaaa...woo-sa-wooo," she said as she humorously imitated her colleague. Hawkinson tried to ignore her, but the performance was too comical. He laughed it up as he smoothly balled up a sheet of paper and tossed it at her. The paper bounced off her forehead and landed in the wastepaper basket next to his desk. Sunflower opened her eyes and laughed it up as well. The two co-workers drifted into a laughing spasm. Every conversation and topic from that point on was hilarious. It had to be. It was that or be consumed by the negative forces outside his office.

*   *   *   *   *

Later on that week just before the Board of Elders, Thadius Powers approached Hawkinson in the milieu. The youth looked a lot healthier since taking a walk on the wild side. He wanted to stand before everyone during the ceremony and apologize for his actions. Hawkinson agreed as he asked everyone to report to the grand room for the Elders ceremony.

After the pledge, Powers was called up to the podium and stood underneath the flags and the three colorful phase banners. His appearance was appropriate. His hygiene was as close to perfection as it was going to get. At first, the youth lowered his head and studied the paper resting on the podium. He cleared his throat about a half dozen times or more before speaking. The room was dead silent.

Powers began reading the apology from the paper. His hands shook nervously. The youth paused in between words and looked at Hawkinson. The Chief Elder pointed to his heart. The youth slowly crumpled the paper and spoke from his heart.

When Powers finished apologizing the room remained silent. He looked around at everyone who was staring at him. He immediately began to heat up and perspire. He lowered his head as he walked back to his seat. Geronimo and Averson stood and slowly began applauding. Soon after, the rest of their peers stood and applauded as well. Never in his life had the youth ever apologized to anyone for his offensive behaviors. The apology was just as foreign as the applause he received.

*   *   *   *   *

After the Elders ceremony, Powers approached Hawkinson. He held out his fist for a pound. Hawkinson smiled and gave the youth a pound in return. His eyes screamed, *I'm sorry for offending you!* Powers made small talk as most people did when they were uncomfortable.

When the youth spotted Sunflower across the room, he started to approach her but instantly stopped. He remembered he was on ban to her for his stalking behaviors and inability to separate his fantasy from reality. The decision was made by the team. The youth walked away and sat alone before pulling out his journal to write down his thought distortions.

The other youth changed out of their dress clothes into Lake Apache sweatsuits and were now enjoying recreation. Hawkinson roved around observing the youth in the milieu. A couple of youth sat in a corner playing their guitars listening to a track by Tom Petty entitled *Free Falling*. A few more youth played cards in the game room while listening to a track by Lupe Fiasco entitled *Superstar*. Another group including Averson, Geronimo and Braylon sat in the library as they spoke about current affairs and politics while listening to a track by Common entitled *Misunderstood*. Hawkinson found himself drawn into the conversation by the youth. He stayed for a while and debated with them. He enjoyed giving input as much as he enjoyed receiving from the young intellects.

While on the way back to his office Hawkinson observed Franklin Roosevelt sitting inside the timeout room. He asked the youth what was going on. He expressed that he needed to get away from everyone and think. He was turning eighteen the next day and he felt a desperate need to make some changes in his life. He discussed the dysfunctional, violent environment in his home. He went into detail about how the criminal actions of family members and others in that environment influenced him heavily. He also discussed his fears of turning out just like them.

Franklin was an intelligent young man with a wealth of insight. A part of him wanted to cut himself off from family members who were consistently involving themselves with criminal actions, but he didn't know how. The youth had never opened up and shared that part of his world with anyone. Like most, he was governed by fear and guilt. The fear and guilt that kept him from letting his greatness shine through. He and Hawkinson conversed for a while. At the end of the conversation, he thanked the counselor that he once defied and despised the most for listening to his thoughts and opinions.

Out in the milieu Hawkinson could sense a difference in the youth. The energy was more calm and peaceful. The noise level was at a minimum. The youth actually shared conversation and debated instead of yelling and hollering at one another. All was well on unit eight, at least for the time being.

Hawkinson returned to his office. It had been a long week. It was the last day before his two days off. He sat down in the chair behind his desk and sighed deeply as he pressed play on the cd player. The lyrics from a track by Will Smith featuring Jill Scott entitled *The Rain* flowed freely from the speakers. He listened to the lyrics. The rain symbolized trying times. Hawkinson had been tried often that week. In fact, it rained so hard it flooded. Trying times covered the land, but Hawkinson stayed afloat in his ark of optimism. The sun shined on him brightly as it always did. When the track ended, he smiled to himself and packed it in for the night before heading home.

*   *   *   *   *

It was Mother's Day when Hawkinson returned from his two days off. It was a day that most of the youth tried to avoid and rightly so. The majority of them didn't want to remember the emotional pain and suffering caused by the absence of the person deemed to be their nurturer, protector and provider. It was much easier to block out mother and forget about her as many had done most of their lives.

During the Men of Distinction group that focused on mothers, the youth were asked to discus in detail something positive or inspirational they remembered most about their mother or mother figure. If there were no positive memories, Hawkinson asked them to create something positive they would say to their mother as if she was there in the room with them.

Most of the youth fidgeted nervously as the anxiety grew. The more emotionally challenged youth rocked and swayed while they chewed nervously at their fingernails. Some of the others leaned their heads to the side.

A couple of the more vocal youth challenged Hawkinson on the assignment. They wanted to know how it would benefit them. Hawkinson explained to the youth that the exercise would help them on an emotional level.

Chapter 19
Mother's Day
(A letter for Momma)

Surprisingly, Franklin began by expressing his most memorable moment about his mother. A track by Boyz II Men entitled *A Song For Mama* played faintly in the background. The youth expressed that when he was about five, he remembered his mother sitting on the edge of a bathtub. He specifically remembered her wearing a tattered robe holding a pipe instrument of some sort up to her lips inhaling deeply. When she noticed him watching her, she kicked the door as it slammed shut in his face. He knocked on the door, but she refused to open it. A tall thin unkept man with poor hygiene approached the door and pushed him aside. He looked at the child with glazed over eyes before entering the bathroom. He then pushed the door shut, but not all the way.

Roosevelt Franklin looked through the crack of the door as he watched his mother and the man take turns inhaling the substance inside the pipe. After they finished smoking, they both exited the bathroom and walked past him like zombies. They entered the bedroom. He watched his mother disrobe. The man performed many beastly acts on her that shattered the child's innocence. He remembered standing there watching, crying and pleading for the man to get away from his mother. The man looked over at him with the same glazed over look and told him to shut up and watch so he could learn what it meant to be a real man.

The room was silent as Franklin continued telling his story. After the first man, came more of them. Sometimes there would be multiple men at one time sharing his mother in sickening ways that no child should ever have to witness. Internally he grew numb from watching the experiences day after day. What was supposed to be a private act of beauty became something demonized as it corrupted the youth's cognitive functioning.

On occasions, some of the men even attempted to incorporate him into the act with his mother, but she fought them off and offered them more of her services. The youth told the group that although his mother was strung out on drugs, she never allowed the men to prey upon him and for that he respected her. A few years later, she walked out with one of those men and never returned. He'd been motherless ever since.

Brennen shared next. The most memorable memory of his mother is when she was a part-time waitress and a full time drunk at a local bar back in his hometown of Louisville. She was hardly ever home so he was forced to raise himself. Brennen was bullied by the school's yuppies, preps and jocks. He told everyone it was because he was dirt poor and lived in a trailer park, which was on the other side of the tracks.

"The kids on the other side of the tracks always got picked on," he said staring intensely at the floor. One day he was on his way home from school with other kids from his trailer park when a group of jocks drove up looking for trouble. He attempted to run but there were too many of them. They chased him down and cornered him. They ripped off his backpack and trashed everything inside before beating him down.

During the time he was being beat, the sound of a horn playing Dixie filled the airwaves. Brennen's mother and a posse of men from the bar pulled up in a pick-up truck. They all jumped out with baseball bats and roughed the jocks up before sending them on their way. The youth expressed that even though he had a deep resentment towards his mother, from that moment on she could do no wrong in his eyes.

Braylon was the next youth to share his most memorable moment of his mother figure. He had an innocent smirk that exposed his chipped tooth. The person he chose to speak about was his older sister. He shared with the group what he'd already shared with Hawkinson about his sister saving him from getting hit by a car. He expressed that Sunflower reminded him a lot of his sister with her humorous and caring ways and that's why he respected her so much. Sunflower was honored as she smiled inside and listened to the youth share his memories.

After sharing comments about his sister, the youth paused and pulled a letter from his journal. He told the group that he wrote a letter to his biological mother and would like to read it to the group which was a quantum leap of improvement for Braylon in treatment. He cleared his throat a half dozen times before reading:

"Dear momma, I wrote this letter for you when I was fourteen. This is your baby boy Braylon aka Bam Bam. Do you remember me, you probably don't, but anyway, every day since I can remember I've thought about you. Every night since I can remember I cried myself to sleep thinking about you. I used to think you left me because you hated me and I was the only boy. When I turned two the first words I ever spoke was momma. I said those words to your oldest daughter. Do you remember her? Probably not, but anyway, I grew up thinking my oldest sister was my momma until I turned five years old. I was told by one of my cousins at my fifth birthday party that the person I was led to believe was my momma was actually my sister. He said I didn't have a momma. I started crying. Can you believe that shit momma, your baby boy was actually crying because he didn't have a momma. For the longest time I didn't want to believe it. My sister confirmed that it was true. I was mad at her and everybody else in the family, but do you know who I was really mad at, if you guessed you then you're damn right. I didn't trust anyone after that, so I hit the streets. One day while I was in the streets a dope head I was selling crack to told me I looked like some older cat named B-nizzle. When I asked what was his last name, he told me Nicholson. Do you remember that name momma, probably not but anyway, I later asked my grandmother, your mother about a guy named B-nizzle Nicholson, you remember your mother, probably not, but anyway she told me what I knew all along. She told me he was my father. Oh shit a father I thought, I didn't even know little ghetto kids like me was supposed to have one of those. Not only was he my father, but he was a crack head, the same crack head who turned you on to crack. She told me you left your family for crack, for drugs. Did you choose drugs over us momma? Did you choose drugs over me? Why momma…why? I just wanted to let you know that my oldest sister is my mother and she did a damn good job raising me, but I let her down by getting locked up, just like you let us down. Maybe I'm just like you momma or maybe… I'm just like that cat who was supposed to be my father. Maybe I have yours and his crack genes. Maybe I ran out on my sisters because you ran out on me. Why you leave us momma? Why you leave? Love your baby boy, aka Bam-Bam B-nizzle."

The room was silent when he finished reading. Some of the youth twitched nervously in their seats. They didn't know how to respond. They'd never listened to Braylon expose himself so candidly.

"I just wanna know why she left me Mr. Hawkinson. I just wanna know why," Braylon said breaking the silence as his bottom lip quivered and a band of tears escaped his ducts. Sunflower rushed out of the room and quickly returned with a box of Kleenex for the teary eyed youth. Some of his peers grew emotional from his emotions, but most grew emotional from the Dear Momma letter, because many of them were in the same predicament. They had no mother either. Hawkinson cautiously walked up behind the youth and placed a healing hand on his shoulder. The youth opened up like a floodgate.

"Why don't she want me Mr. Hawk? Why don't my momma want me?" Braylon continued to ask as the tears flowed and his voice cracked. Hawkinson kept his hand on the youth's shoulder. The box of Kleenex circulated around the room. Every youth was wiping his eyes and blowing his nose. Even a couple of the staff temporarily exited the room to escape the moment. Through all the sniffling and tear shedding, Braylon's peers developed a newfound respect for him. He was always respected because of his sharp wit and physical dominance, but now he was respected even more. The youth showed courage by doing something none of his peers had the courage to do and that was exposing a more passionate, intelligent side of his nature by crying instead of fighting. He was highly honored by his peers for that.

LaBoy stood and approached Braylon. He held out a hand and shared with Braylon that he had no mother either. She died a few years ago from an illness. Braylon looked up at LaBoy partially blinded by his tears. He slowly stood. The two youth embraced one another awkwardly as they shed more tears. Geronimo, Brennen, Roosevelt and Averson approached the two and joined in the embrace. Pretty soon all the youth were on their feet and attached as part of the supportive circle. Sunflower approached Hawkinson and stood next to him.

"I can't stand you Hawk— got me all moist in the eyes. You know I don't like showing emotions here. No one else could have pulled this off but you," she said playfully elbowing her colleague as she wiped a runaway tear from her face. He stuck out his fist for a pound. Sunflower gave him a pound in return. Watching all the male youth bond and support one another was a sight to see. A few months ago, Braylon and LaBoy were enemies to the death, now they were comrades on the battlefield of emotions supporting one another.

The recovery phase focused on relapse prevention and healing, and there was a lot of healing going on at that particular moment. After the youth finished supporting one another they returned to their seats. Hawkinson asked by show of hands how many of the youth would like to write a letter to their alive or deceased mother. Every hand in the room went into the air. Hawkinson had the shredder waiting on standby for those who didn't want to mail the letter, but just wanted to relieve bottled up feelings and emotions.

The youth opened their journals and proceeded to write. Playing faintly in the background was a song by Kanye West entitled *Hey Mama.* The youth sat quietly as their deepest emotions guided the pens that produced black ink across the smoothness of the white paper. Some shed tears as they wrote. Others frowned, sighed deeply and crumpled sheets of paper. Hawkinson could feel the mental energy transpired by feelings and emotions moving all around him.

*　　*　　*　　*　　*

After the writing session, some kept the letters to mama while others took advantage of the shredder. There was an uncomfortable silence that governed the room. For many, silence was scary and fearful. Something extremely powerful had just occurred and they didn't know how to approach it. Hawkinson could see a few of the youth growing antsy. Before the fidgety behaviors had a chance to grow into a monster of uncontrolled emotions, Hawkinson explained the power of silence to the youth. He reminded them of the silence after the meditation period while encouraging them to return to that blissful moment.

Geronimo, Averson, Franklin, Sanchez and a few others closed their eyes and breathed deeply until they were relaxed and one with the silence. Right before his very eyes, Hawkinson could see the worry and fretfulness melt away from their being. When they returned from the ocean of silence their eyes were bright and focused. The fear and anxiety that once existed no longer resided.

*　　*　　*　　*　　*

Later that afternoon in the dining hall as the youth feasted away on a special Mother's Day meal, Braylon sat alone staring out into nothingness. Hawkinson approached the youth and asked if he could join him. The youth stood and welcomed Hawkinson who sat. Braylon sat down beside him. The senior counselor took notice of Braylon's mannerisms.

"I appreciate the courtesy you just displayed. How come you're not eating?"

"I learned from a wise one that a true warrior always eats last. He displays gratitude and appreciation to the others by allowing them to eat before him. It's a part of giving back. When I first took notice of you doing that Mr. Hawkinson, I thought it was a sign of weakness. Nobody ever cared if I ate first in the world that I came from."

"And no one probably will in the world that you return to, but it will do wonders for your character. Have you been spying on me youth Braylon?"

"No sir, just watching closely. We all watch you. We watch everything you do. The way you walk straight as an arrow with your spine erect and feet barely touching the ground. We watch the way you greet people with a golden smile. The way you open and hold doors for others. We even watch the way you treat the women around campus with respect. Where I'm from the goons talk down to women. You also treat us youth with respect. Even when you're disciplining us the majority knows it's out of care and concern. You don't talk down to us like we're nothing. You treat us like we're somebody."

"You are somebody and don't you ever let anyone tell you differently."

"We're youth offenders Mr. Hawkinson."

"No, you're youth that have committed offenses against others and yourself. You have the power to correct that. Until you forgive yourself and start to love yourself, you'll continue to offend others while wearing that offensive label." Hawkinson asked Braylon if anyone ever told him that he was bad while growing up. The youth responded by nodding his head yes. He explained to the youth if an individual is told he or she is something long enough, they start to believe in those words and take on that particular personality. He told Braylon that words carry power. He also told him that he believed there is no such thing as bad children. Children are a boundless energy of love that happen to conform to the environment that they're in. If it's a violent, uncivilized environment, then more than likely that's what the child will conform to. If it's an environment of love, peace, harmony, knowledge, wisdom and self-respect, the child has a greater chance of conforming to that and becoming successful in life. Braylon pondered upon Hawkinson's words of advice as he always did.

"So that's why you always say we are a product of our environment."

"That's what we are, conformists…but you have the power to change that."

"Youth Geronimo told me treatment is a blessing in disguise. He said he used to have dreams that he would come here. He said he was destined to come here, to meet you."

"What do you think?"

"At first I thought he had been secretly sneaking in the cleaning closet sniffing chemicals," the youth said with an honest expression. Hawkinson chuckled at his response.

"But, after I observed you for myself and took notice of your consistent actions, I became a believer."

Hawkinson asked the youth what he currently thought about being at Lake Apache. Braylon told Hawkinson he always wanted to be in an environment where he could learn and get away from the hustle of the street life. He had dreams about coming to a place like Lake Apache when he was in corrections. He expressed that it was scary because he thought he was going to die in corrections and the dreams of Lake Apache was his afterlife.

Hawkinson expressed to Braylon that the lesser part of him has died and the greater part of him has been resurrected. The youth sat quietly and reflected.

Braylon had worked diligently at catching up on his treatment assignments. He was the first youth ever to have left the academy and return to catch up on his assignments while staying on target to graduate.

Hawkinson shared with the youth how proud he was of him. The two conversed a while longer about how much Braylon had grown since the Thanksgiving feast when he sat in the same spot with a much different attitude. After everyone had gone through the meal line, Hawkinson and Braylon approached to get a meal. Mother's Day turned out to be a great day. The youth of Lake Apache Academy had a different outlook on the most underrated holiday on the twelve month calendar.

Chapter 20

Testimonial Confessions of a Youth Offender

It was mid May. The anticipation of graduation, which was two months away was starting to take its toll on the youth and staff. Many youth rushed to complete past due assignments. LaBoy was one of those youth. He was far behind in his treatment work. Braylon stepped up to help the youth out just as Geronimo and Averson once helped him.

Powers continued to struggle with his ban to Sunflower. He found any little excuse to try and make conversation with her. His creepy, stalking behaviors didn't go unnoticed by his peers. They were right there each time to hold him accountable. Due to the incident he had on the day of the cookout, Powers was on a short leash with his parole agent. One more incident on that level and he was guaranteed a trip back to the Department of Corrections. The youth knew just how far to take it. He would make certain comments or perform certain behaviors and pull out of the action just before it warranted a consequence.

None of his peers wanted to be around him and most of the staff grew tired of him. The mental sickness that resided within him seemed to spawn. The clinical team chose to have him diagnosed by the campus psychologist. Powers received a medication change to help take the manic aggressive edge off. It would take a few days for changes to kick in. Meanwhile, the team observed him closely.

Averson met with Hawkinson for an individual session. During the session he discussed his poor relationship with his biological parents. He blamed most of his delinquent behaviors for their absence early on in life. Averson discussed being an only child and not having anyone to confide in.

The family that took him in at a young age were extremely wealthy. He expressed that he always felt as if he was a replacement for their son who'd gone away to college. They gave him everything he wanted without challenging him. When he got into trouble at school, they made excuses for his behaviors. When he intentionally broke things in the home they replaced it without questioning his actions. The foster parents ignored his cry for attention and love.

The youth decided that when he entered junior high he would turn it up a few notches. He began hanging around an older high school crowd. He snuck out of the house late at night and went joy riding. He crashed parties that served plenty of alcohol, drugs and sex. That's when his substance abuse issues began. Surely the foster parents would pay attention to him now, at least that's what he thought. Instead, they took him to see a psychiatrist believing that would solve everything. Averson admitted to delving deeper into drugs. He smoked as much marijuana as he could to block out what was going on around him and to numb what he was feeling deep inside. When the temporary high wore off his problems increased even more.

When the foster family could no longer put up with his disruptive behaviors, they asked that he be removed from their home. From that point, Averson's issues worsened. He continued to get into trouble with the law. He said his primary issue was rejection. His world finally came crashing down when he was caught stealing to support his nicotine and narcotic habits. Due to his mile long rap sheet, the judge and public defender thought it would be best if the youth served some time in a juvenile detention center before attending a boot camp. After serving time, he was released. Instead of a boot camp, the judge ordered him to attend Lake Apache Academy for an intense, eleven month treatment program.

Averson confessed that he feared being locked up. He had to watch his back everyday. If someone wasn't trying to take his food, they were stealing his hygiene products and then trying to sell them back to him. When they weren't trying to steal his products they were trying to steal his manhood. For the first time ever he found himself physically fighting for his life everyday. The fighting extended his time. Six months turned into nine, and nine into twelve.

"What made you continue fighting?" Hawkinson asked.

"I had to prove I wasn't a punk bitch, especially being a white kid from the suburbs," the youth said clenching his teeth together as if he was reliving the moment.

In between the youth telling his DOC war stories, Hawkinson complimented him on his health. He'd lost weight and his overall demeanor appeared more confident unlike when he first arrived at the academy back in the late summer. The youth smiled bashfully as he continued his testimony. The challenging part of his treatment was to recover from the emotional trauma. It was time to discard the unhealthy behaviors and replace them with healthy ones.

*   *   *   *   *

Later that week Hawkinson met with Geronimo. During past sessions the youth had been compliant, humble and open. As the sessions progressed and intensified, he began to shut down and grow more standoffish. His demeanor expressed that he didn't want to be there. He purposely skipped hair cut day and it showed. His frizzy hair was starting to grow out of control like a chia pet. The depressed youth pulled the hood of his hoodie over his head. Earlier that day he'd gotten into two verbal altercations that nearly turned physical. When Hawkinson asked where he was in his anger cycle, the youth shrugged his shoulders.

"Okay, okay," the senior staff said silencing himself. Something he learned over the past cycles as a therapeutic counselor was to never work harder than the client. If he found himself working harder than the client, there was no therapy taking place. He sat in silence reading a Scientific International Mind magazine. Geronimo sighed deeply as if he was trying to get his attention. Hawkinson peered over the magazine and raised his right eyebrow as he always did.

"You need something?" he asked the youth.

"Just clearing my throat," he said.

"Okay," Hawkinson said as he went back to reading his magazine. The youth continued clearing his throat. Hawkinson sat the magazine down and focused his attention on Geronimo. He challenged the youth by asking him to speak the first thing that entered his mind after he asked him a question.

"Who hurt you?" he asked the youth. Geronimo's eyes dropped as he answered the question immediately. He shared that he was hurt by his mother, who abandoned him by running off with her girlfriend when he was a young child. His foster dad attempted to beat the sins of life out of him while beating religion into him.

When he grew older, Geronimo went searching for his biological father who was wealthy, remarried and living in the northern suburbs of Chicago with his new family. His father recognized him the moment he opened the door and made eye contact. He invited the youth in and had a long talk with him. He mostly conversed about the life between he and the youth's mother before Geronimo was born. No love was shared from the father or apology given for not being a part of his life. After the conversation, his father drove him back to the city, placed a hefty wad of cash in his hand and told him it would be best if he didn't come to see him or his family anymore.

The youth told Hawkinson he took the cash and exited the car. As the man he called his father drove away, he cursed him in his thoughts and washed his hands free of him, wishing he'd die on the freeway from an accident while traveling back to his suburban home. Geronimo caught a bus downtown where he often went to converse with the homeless. He found refuge in their conversation. It was his safe harbor. He used the cash from the man he no longer identified as his father to buy food and clothing for a homeless man he befriended.

Geronimo told Hawkinson he confided in the homeless man who once lived his life as a successful wealthy man. The homeless man didn't judge him and he didn't judge the homeless man. He told Hawkinson that the foster father came looking for him. When he found Geronimo, he threatened to whip him with his infamous leather strap if he ever returned to the site where the homeless dwelled.

Geronimo returned to the foster home. That evening he refused to go to worship, which took place at least six days out of the week. The youth had been to five of the services that week and didn't want to miss his martial arts competition. The foster father denied him of the competition. When the youth rebelled, the foster father retrieved his strap and commenced to beating the youth. Geronimo had taken several beatings before but this would be the last one. He blocked the next incoming blow and wrapped the strap around his hand before snatching it away. The foster father bull rushed him, but Geronimo was too quick. He used his martial arts skills and side stepped the aggressive man. He crashed hard into an antique China cabinet and cut himself up badly, which left him crippled. The foster father pressed charges and told the arresting officer and the courts that the youth threw him into the cabinet. Geronimo was charged and arrested before he was sent away to corrections.

"You didn't throw him into the cabinet as the reports claim, did you?" Hawkinson asked in a supportive tone.

"No sir, I never touched him. Since then I've spent time in a place not suitable for me. I often questioned myself....Was I that bad to have the things happen to me that were happening... or was it something I did in a past life?" the youth said swallowing deeply as the tears began to well up.

"Why didn't you dispute the charge?"

"Because, I figured the hell I was heading for had to be a step up from the one I'd just left."

"Okay, okay," Hawkinson said in a comforting tone as he guided his index finger across his forehead to the center of his third eye. He stroked the center of his frontal lobe before allowing his finger to trace down the bridge of his nose and rest on his upper lip. Okay was his signature word and the stroking of the frontal lobe was his signature move when he was either thinking deeply or faced with a challenging task.

The youth sat quietly and gathered himself before continuing. He went into his memory museum and discussed things that were done to him that would make the average human cringe. Hawkinson struggled to understand how the youth was even functioning at such a high level of intelligence after such horrid events.

After the session was over Hawkinson needed to get outdoors for a while for some self-care. He embraced the sunrays and the other unseen elements as he quieted his mind to meditate. The purpose of meditating was to clear his mind and slow his thought process. Meditation allowed him to relieve the dense stress energy and tension accumulated throughout the day from others' darkened energy. To successfully treat clients, Hawkinson always made sure he first treated his own mind, body and spirit. As a practitioner he allowed the universal force of perfect intelligence to govern his mental activity. He also saw each client as a perfect divine creation of the sum of all.

When Hawkinson returned from his treatment hour, he felt mentally energized and rejuvenated. He was prepared for the challenges to come. Sunflower appeared at the door. She was holding a sheet of paper with information written on it.

"Hey grasshopper, while you were out doing your woo-sa stress reliever thing you had a phone call from a past client. He said it was urgent that he speaks with you," she said entering and handing the information to him. Hawkinson read the name and phone number on the paper. He immediately recognized the client. He picked up the phone to dial the number. Before he dialed, he looked up at Sunflower who was standing before him pretending to sift through a stack of papers.

"Thank you. I can handle it from here," he said shifting his eyes towards the door.

"Hawk, are you implying that I'm trying to listen to your conversation. If so, I am really disappointed in you," she said turning to leave while taking her time.

"As you're picking up that nosey pace, please close the door behind you," he said as she exited the office.

"Whatever Hawk," Sunflower chuckled as she closed the door. Sunflower was observant as well as aware as a night owl. She heard and saw everything. Her hearing and visual radars were as sharp as a tack. Hawkinson treasured that about his colleague. It was a strength needed in that field of work.

Hawkinson dialed the number on the paper. The phone rang a few times before a depressed tone of voice answered. When Hawkinson greeted the young man on the other end, he perked up. The two of them shared conversation about his most recent successes and failures. Judging by the nature of his conversation the young man was struggling greatly. Hawkinson listened with a sound ear. When the former youth finished sharing about his short stay in jail along with being a new father, Hawkinson offered his support. Afterwards, he hung up the phone and sighed deeply. Seconds later Sunflower burst through the door.

"Okay Hawk, give me the 411 on when he got out of jail and who did he get pregnant?"

"Maya! There's just no end to your blooming curiosity, is it?"

"You have to learn to talk a little lower Hawk. You have a problem with your voice escalation," she said chuckling. "Now stop stalling and give me the 411." Hawkinson could only shake his head at his inquisitive co-worker.

*   *   *   *   *

Hawkinson entered the relaxation group. The youth were all waiting patiently. They seemed eager to get started. The group began with a brief discussion of what took place in the last relaxation group. Hawkinson was impressed. In this particular group, the goal was to focus more on deep breathing while creating through visual imagery. Hawkinson began the background music, which was Native American flutes and irish bag pipes. The youth closed their eyes and began a pattern of deep breathing as they had been instructed to do.

After about ninety seconds into the deep breathing, Hawkinson's baritone voice infiltrated their world. The first word to roll off his tongue was love. He repeated the word love twelve more times before giving the visual location. In the visual he asked the youth to strap on their wings. He then flew them far off to a doorway carved into a large vertical plate of rock. The door had a heart-shaped indention in the middle of it. After he had each of them align their hearts with the heart in the door, he instructed them to touch the door.

When the youth touched the door in their visual it slowly opened. On the other side of the door was a beautiful lake. In the middle of the lake he described an island. The island was made of red rock similar to the red rock in New Mexico and Arizona. The landscaping was breathtaking.

Hawkinson instructed the youth to fly over the lake to the island. Once they were on the island he appointed each of them to take their place upon a throne made of the exact same red rock that surrounded the island. In the vision he described the rock as solar rock made of the same powerful radiation and elements of the central sun in our current galaxy, which gives life to the sun that illuminates the planet earth. Hawkinson went on to explain that near the nape of their necks, close to their medulla oblongata was a blue stone embedded in the red rock. The stone resembled a mirror. The purpose of the stone was to bore out the negative images the youth had accumulated in their thought process. He asked the youth to feel the energy and the vibration rushing up from their feet to their legs up the back of their spines to the center of their hearts and up to the center of their third eye.

After the youth did what was asked of them in their vision, Hawkinson repeated the word love thirteen more times. He explained that the energy they felt rushing through their feet from the red rock through the rest of their being was love. It was the pure cosmic force straight from the source of all existence.

Hawkinson then asked the youth to begin shedding and peeling away the layers of anger, disappointment, hate and any other ill feelings they'd been harboring. With every word Hawkinson spoke to the youth, he could see their physical demeanor loosen up as they slumped down into their chairs. For the next several minutes, he allowed the youth to go through this healing process.

After a period of time elapsed, Hawkinson slowly and carefully returned the youth from the thrones, off the island, across the lake through the rock door, across the clear blue skies, back to Lake Apache into the group room and onto the chairs. He allowed the youth to gather themselves before processing their experience.

*   *   *   *   *

When the seven youth exited the group, smiling and stepping as if they walked on water, their peers stared at them in amazement.

"Whoa, check them out," one youth said to the others. Everyone wanted to know why the seven youth looked so carefree and brand new. They followed them around inquiring about their experiences during the relaxation group. Averson told his peers it was the best drug free high he ever experienced.

Chapter 21
Righting the Wrongs
(Paying it Forward)

One of the main assignments for the youth on the blue phase was to give back by volunteering their services to local businesses. Giving back helped the youth prepare for the empathy assignment. It taught them that giving from the heart and soul without asking for anything in return expressed a humanitarian effort. Interacting with the elderly at a local nursing home, cleaning the streets each night of a 3-day festival in town, painting the walls of local businesses, picking up trash along sidewalks and feeding the homeless at a local Salvation Army were the volunteer assignments offered to the youth.

Many of the youth had never offered charitable contributions to anyone. All they knew was to take from others. Most felt as though the world owed them something. Hawkinson explained that offering their volunteer services to others would help right their wrongs. The youth complained that giving back to a group of strangers they never met seemed odd. Hawkinson asked if it felt odd when they took from strangers and others they didn't know. The room grew dead silent.

The youth were split up into five groups of five. The first group, which consisted of Braylon and four other youth, awoke at 4:00 a.m. to go to the local town and clean the streets after a festival. Hawkinson supervised the youth. The streets were full of debris. The beer tents were a weakness for the youth with past alcohol abuse issues. Braylon who could not stand the smell of the alcohol stained tables and half filled cups of beer, cleaned the tents quickly and encouraged his peers to do the same.

Hawkinson helped the youth with their cleaning duties. He worked just as diligently as they did. His leadership alone motivated them to work more consistently. He was their example. When the youth finished, they looked at the area they cleaned and gave each other high fives. They covered at least four blocks of cleaning, sweeping and using a blower to blow the trash in the middle of the streets for the street sweeper. Hawkinson told them he was proud of the work they'd done.

When the youth returned to campus they boasted about their experience as volunteers. Their energy seemed to motivate some of the others who hadn't yet volunteered their services. A group was held and the five youth whom already had the experience openly spoke before the rest of their peers. The first youth shared how tempting it was for him to be in the vicinity with the tents that served alcohol. He expressed that all of his past issues with alcoholic parents and abusing alcohol himself affected him greatly the first couple of days. By the third day, he admitted that he actually grew disgusted by the smell of cigarette butts floating in the cups of the leftover alcohol.

The second youth discussed the environment itself being a set up for him. The youth had a history of drinking, smoking and stealing everything he touched. His biggest struggle was when he found a wallet lying on the ground near a vendors booth. The wallet was full of cash and had credit cards in it as well. The youth said he first kicked the wallet under a pile of trash while he was sweeping so that no one could see it. He amitted when Hawkinson turned his head to observe one of the other youth, he quickly reached down and picked up the wallet before stuffing it in his pants. He went back to cleaning before the guilt and paranoia slowly began to eat away at him from the inside out. The youth expressed that whenever Hawkinson would look through him with those piercing eyes, he perspired profusely. The guilt knots in his stomach allowed him to surrender the wallet over to Hawkinson.

Braylon expressed that at first he didn't understand the concept of giving back and only volunteered his charitable services because it was what he had to do on the recovery phase to graduate. After the second day, some of the town officials drove up and commended him and his peers for the outstanding work they were doing. One of the officials told Braylon he'd been observing him and appreciated his dedication and leadership. He handed him a business card with the number to his establishment and told him if he ever needed a job to give him a call.

Braylon expressed that it was at that moment he realized he made a difference in someone else's life and someone other than Hawkinson appreciated his strengths. He admitted it felt good. He felt appreciated. It made him want to work even harder on the last day.

*   *   *   *   *

The next group to volunteer their charitable services was youth Geronimo, Franklin and three other peers. Minnis supervised the five youth cutting the lawns of the elderly in the nearby town. A couple of the youth had never operated a lawnmower or weed whacker. Minnis had them pair up with the more skilled lawn cutters. Youth Roosevelt was a hard worker. He cut the grass and trimmed the weeds consistently. Every so often he complained about the sun's intensity but he continued to work. Geronimo wasn't a grass cutter, but he was able to manage the mower and do a pretty good job due to his personality and overall work ethic. He and Franklin showed great leadership.

*   *   *   *   *

Hawkinson met with Roosevelt Franklin for an individual session later that evening. The youth began the session by discussing his persoanl changes since his eighteenth birthday. Hawkinson could see a great change in the youth's attitude. He appeared more humble and more knowledgable since the first day he arrived. His hair was cut and groomed. His pants no longer sagged below his waistline. The nicotine itch he used to have was still there, but he managed it a lot better. Foul words of aggression no longer rolled off his tongue polluting his surroundings. The youth was definitely a changed individual.

Franklin compared his past marijuana abuse to the relaxation and meditation. He told Hawkinson he used to get high every day since the age of eleven, but that type of high couldn't compare to the relaxation group. He admitted to being afraid and skeptical when he first tried the meditation. The results made him more calm and less paranoid unlike the marijuana. He focused more on his classroom and treatment assignments. His confidence level grew.

The youth directed his focus to a large colorful painting hanging on the wall with a symbolic calendar next to it. It was something he'd been studying since he first visited Hawkinson's office. Hawkinson asked him if he knew what the portrait symbolized. The youth shook his head no as he continued to study the intricate designs and colors in the portrait.

Hawkinson explained that the symbol is known as the tree of life. According to the Mayan philosophy, the tree is the source of all life including human beings. It is a tree that has turned this earth into a living vibrating world where everything is connected and co-dependent.

"The man in the center of the portrait is sinking into the tree later to be reborn as its branches," explained Hawkinson.

Franklin studied the art even closer. He asked what the funny looking calendar symbolized. Hawkinson explained that it was the Mayan calendar which shares its messages or symbols as spiritual traditions. A few of the Mayan traditions have branched out and touched the world. Hawkinson explained, "We are all one, life has a purpose and most importantly, God is love. Those are the three messages. Winter solstice 2012 marks the end of this historical calendar."

The youth continued to study the calendar as he asked questions about the symbols and the glyphs. Hawkinson observed the sparkling inquisitiveness in the child's eyes. Roosevelt Franklin was a seed waiting to be watered and fed so that he could sprout, grow and evolve.

*   *   *   *   *

Hawkinson returned to work after two days off. He met with the rest of the team for a briefing before taking to the milieu. Sunflower asked about his weekend. He told her about multiple graduation celebrations he attended.

"You're such a good role model Hawk. I'm so proud of you," she said patting him on the back.

"I'll be proud of you too if you can get first place in the staff physical performance test this week. I hope you're ready."

"Please, I was born ready," she scoffed.

"We'll see when you're inhaling my dust," he chuckled.

"It's not a race Hawk. It's a physical performance test. You are so competitive," she said walking away.

*   *   *   *   *

Later that morning, Hawkinson and Sunflower drove the third of the fifth group to a home for senior citizens. The plan was for the five youth to volunteer their services by socializing with the seniors before serving them for afternoon lunch. The youth appeared timid when they arrived at the home.

A nurse gave them a tour and introduced them to several of the seniors. A couple of the youth took to the seniors right away by sitting and playing a game of cards. The other three sat back and observed their surroundings while waiting for the seniors to approach them. Right away Hawkinson could tell which of the youth had social skills and which ones didn't. One very humorous senior pointed to the three youth sitting back and engaged them.

"Hey you lil' three crumb snatching snap dragons, get on over here so I can absorb the wetness dripping from behind your ears with this here deck of cards," he chuckled. LaBoy and the other two youth looked at each other and chuckled.

"Yeah I'm talking to you Bones, Thugs and Disharmony. You tough guys aren't scared are you?" he asked pointing and purposely slipping his dentures in and out of his mouth while wiggling his eyebrows. Two of the youth accepted the challenge.

LaBoy sat back observing everyone. Hawkinson approached and asked the youth why wasn't he interacting. LaBoy sighed before speaking. He expressed that he was having mixed emotions. A part of him felt sorry for the seniors that suffered from chronic pain and other ailments. He also expressed that some of them were humorous as they sat around roasting and arguing amongst one another. He told Hawkinson they reminded him of the elderly gentlemen back on his block who sat around all day exchanging sips from a brown paper bag telling stories about the good old days.

Hawkinson listened imaginatively to what the youth was describing. He then encouraged LaBoy to go over and introduce himself to the seniors. The youth stood and approached a group of seniors sitting around a table playing Poker. They welcomed him and encouraged him to partake in the game. He opted to watch. LaBoy looked up and spotted an elderly woman sitting in a corner of the room by herself. She was staring directly at him. He looked away but at times he found himself locking eyes with the woman. Hawkinson watched LaBoy's interactions. He also noticed how the elderly woman continued to stare at him.

During lunch, the five youth had grown somewhat accustomed to the seniors. They were happy to serve them as they stood behind the food line wearing their plastic gloves and hairnets. The seniors were grateful to the youth for spending the morning and afternoon with them. After lunch the youth cleaned up before saying their goodbyes.

*　　*　　*　　*　　*

Later that week Hawkinson met with LaBoy for an individual therapy session. The youth began the session discussing a phone call he had with his father that turned into an ugly argument. All of LaBoy's phone calls with his father ended in a yelling match or some type of disagreement. Hawkinson realized why LaBoy was the way he was. The fruit didn't fall too far from the tree. In this case it could have easly been an acorn. The youth was the spitting image of his father, but of course he didn't recognize the similarities he shared with LaBoy Sr.

There was no talking to LaBoy Sr. once he got going. Hawkinson tried several times to engage him in telephone conversations. Everything was everyone else's fault. There was no self-accountability. LaBoy Sr. is what Hawkinson likes to refer to as a spindoctor driving in a victim mobile. He tried to rotate and project every negative thing that took place in his life onto his son, Hawkinson and the other Lake Apache staff. He was a victim of his own projecting distorted thoughts.

Hawkinson asked the youth how he prepared to get along with his father since he would be returning to his home after he graduated treatment. The youth shrugged his shoulders in a hopeless manner. Hawkinson suggested that his father come to the academy for family sessions once a week for the next six weeks. LaBoy sighed and expressed that his father wouldn't participate due to lack of transportation. The persistent counselor explained that the academy would provide transportation between the Metra train station and the facility.

Hawkinson called the youth's father to set up a family session with the family therapist who had no luck in getting LaBoy Sr. to attend sessions. He came up with every excuse under the sun to not attend the session, but the crafty Hawkinson had a resolution for the excuses. He was somehow able to get LaBoy Sr. to attend the sessions. LaBoy Sr. attempted to morph into his role as spindoctor, but Hawkinson didn't give him a chance. He cut the conversation short by ending the phone call.

The therapy session resumed. Hawkinson had been waiting to ask the youth a question about a situation he observed at the senior citizens home earlier that week. He asked why was he staring at the elderly woman who couldn't seem to stop staring at him as well. LaBoy lowered his head and stared at his feet. Hawkinson waited patiently for an answer.

After allowing the question to marinate in his thought process, LaBoy answered. He told Hawkinson a couple of years ago he was out and about in the city after ditching school. He'd been smoking marijuana and drinking with other delinquent dropouts. When the crew ran out of drugs and alcohol they selected LaBoy to replenish their source.

The youth hit the streets under the influence of the substances. He was high which meant he took on a bold character. He stumbled upon the path of a few seniors leaving a supermarket. Without giving it a second thought he ran up to them and snatched a couple of purses. One of the senior women put up a fight as she held on to her purse. LaBoy looked her in the eye. He may have been high, but he remembered the frightened helpless look in her eyes as she stared through his soul. He snatched harder until the strap broke away from her shoulder. The youth tucked the purses under his arm and ran until he was out of breath. He took the money from the purses and tossed them into a dumpster.

He bought more liquor and drugs for his hoods as they sat around listening to him boast about how he robbed the seniors. Youth LaBoy expressed when the high went away, so did his false courage. He couldn't stop thinking about the eyes of the woman piercing through him. He admitted that he thought about the scenario continuously for several weeks. He looked at Hawkinson and sighed.

"I was wrong for what I did, and if I could take it all back… I would."

"What do you do now since you've revealed the phantom?"

"What do you mean?" LaBoy asked.

"Are you prepared to right your wrongs?"

"I feel I need to, but I don't know how." LaBoy sat in silence as he waited for Hawkinson to come up with a plan to rescue him. Every so often he would peer up at the counselor to see what he was doing. Hawkinson was a very wealthy man in the silence and patience department. He sat quietly staring at the youth without blinking. After awhile the buzzer went off. The session was over. In his mind, LaBoy felt as though he escaped the question of how to right his wrongs. He stood to leave.

"Youth LaBoy, I'd like for you to have an answer to the question before we return to the senior citizens home next Sunday for the last visit. Please don't seek out others for help. It was your past doing so that makes it your present assignment. I'll see you later," Hawkinson said to the youth before he exited the office.

Chapter 22
Figures of our Fathers

It was the following Sunday. That morning Hawkinson and Sunflower drove the five youth including LaBoy, back to the senior citizens home. It was a very uncomfortable visit for LaBoy who was quiet during the entire drive. He perspired heavily.

"Calm down big boy, you act like we're going to church for your funeral. You must have lost a good twenty pounds the way you're back there sweating," the humorous youth Brennen said in his southern accent. The other peers took notice of LaBoy's excessive sweating and chuckled while making remarks to one another about his biological condition.

When they reached the site, LaBoy was the last youth to exit the van. He drug his feet as if he was shackled with iron chains on his way to the death chamber. His nerves were tightly knotted. His hands trembled. When they entered the day area, the seniors were happily awaiting them. LaBoy's eyes darted around the room in search of the elderly woman. He sat down at an empty table. His heart felt as if it beat in his throat. Every little noise intensified as it echoed in his ear canal.

Hawkinson appeared behind the youth and placed a calming hand on his shoulder. LaBoy's spirit nearly leaped through the seven layers of his flesh. He looked up at Hawkinson with fearful eyes.

"You ready to right your wrong?"

"Not really, but it's my wrong to right," the youth said wiping the sweat from his brow with his free hand. Hawkinson removed his hand from LaBoy's shoulder as he walked away and approached the nurse in charge for that shift. LaBoy watched from the corner of his eye as Hawkinson and the female staff exchanged conversation before shifting their gaze to him. The already nervous youth swallowed deeply. Never in his life had he felt so nervous and anxious. Although he practiced what he was going to say that entire week, he had no idea how it was going to come out. He was at a loss for words.

Hawkinson and the nurse began walking in his direction. It was as if they were walking in slow motion. Whenever their feet struck the floor, LaBoy felt his heart get ready to blast from his chest. When the two approached, LaBoy was in some sort of daze. The nurse began to speak to him, but her words seemed muffled, that is until LaBoy heard the words *passed away* seep from between her lips. He quickly snapped out of his daze.

"Excuse me ma'am, but can you repeat that?" he asked standing. The nurse repeated her statement. She told LaBoy the elderly woman he sought out passed away last Monday after they visited the nursing home on Sunday. She told LaBoy and Hawkinson that the woman was her great aunt. She moved her to the nursing home from the city a couple of years back after she fell and broke her hip. LaBoy asked how she broke her hip. She told him that her aunt was pushed down to the ground while being mugged by a teenage thug. Hawkinson watched as LaBoy's entire demeanor shifted. His knees buckled. His eyes went dim as if the life force had been driven out of him.

The youth sat down. The flowers he'd been holding for the elderly woman fell from his hands onto the floor. He hung his head and rocked back and forth. The nurse looked from LaBoy to Hawkinson in a confused manner.

"Excuse me, but am I missing something?" she asked. Hawkinson pulled her aside and told her that LaBoy had a connection with her great aunt and was really looking forward to giving her the flowers as well as saying some kind words to her. The nurse smiled. She told Hawkinson that her aunt was buried in the cemetery about a quarter of a mile up the road and LaBoy had her blessings to go and visit the gravesite.

Hawkinson approached the youth and asked if he would like to visit the gravesite. With red watery eyes, he looked up and nodded his head yes. Hawkinson explained to Sunflower what was taking place. She told him that the other youth would be fine until he and LaBoy returned.

Hawkinson and LaBoy walked a quarter of a mile up the road to the graveyard. When they reached the gates, they followed the directions the nurse gave them to her aunt's headstone. When they reached the headstone, Hawkinson gave LaBoy the personal space he needed.

The timid youth approached the gravestone with trembling hands. He cautiously laid the flowers on the ground. He read the name on the gravestone.

The woman's name was Betty Alexandria Foster. LaBoy removed a note from his pocket keeping his eyes on the gravestone the entire time as if something was going to jump out at him. The guilt and fear was eating him from the inside out. He began reading from the note. Shortly into reading, he stopped and balled the letter up and put it back into his pocket.

The youth spoke from his heart. He began by giving Betty's spirit a brief lesson of his history. He talked to the gravestone as if she was actually there standing before him. He discussed the death of his mother and how much he missed her. He also discussed the rotten relationship he has with his father. He then discussed all the great people he met at Lake Apache Academy and how much they have supported and helped him make positive changes in his life. He told Betty he wished he could have gotten to know her better on a personal level.

The youth grew silent. Without any warning, he broke down like the New Orleans levies during hurricane Katrina. The youth fell down to the ground on both knees sobbing uncontrollably. Through all the sniffling and gasping, LaBoy apologized to the deceased woman's gravestone repeatedly for victimizing her. Hawkinson stood back but was on standby in case the youth needed support.

Hawkinson never allowed his emotions to mix with anyone else's. His emotions were his only and when he needed to express them he did. Just like an oak tree planted by water, Hawkinson was not moved. He was a rock as he stood silently with his hands resting behind his back and his head slightly bowed. The emotions LaBoy was experiencing were brought about through his own wrongdoings.

The youth cried out all the hurt and pain he ever projected onto others and the hurt and pain others projected onto him. The emotional bellows were coming from deep within his soul. The average person may have thought the youth was going through some sort of exorcism from the noises that came from within, but Hawkinson knew it was years of built up hurt, anger, guilt, fear and pain. He was crying out for a healing.

LaBoy continued to cry and heal from within as he kneeled before the gravesite. He wiped his eyes and placed his right tear drenched hand on the headstone. A gust of warm wind stirred and swept through the trees in the cemetery. The wind spiraled down and encircled LaBoy embracing him, before washing over Hawkinson and back up to the trees. The wind blew for a while longer before all was settled once again.

"Did you feel that?" the fearful youth asked as he looked over his shoulder at Hawkinson.

"I felt it. She forgives you. Miss Betty Alexandria Foster forgives you and she's moved on to the other side," Hawkinson said embracing the spiritual moment. The floodgates opened even more as tears streamed from the youth's eyes. He turned his head away from Hawkinson in an embarrassing manner.

"It's okay son. Real men do cry, and don't ever let anyone tell you anything different." On that afternoon, LaBoy cried a river. He and Hawkinson walked back to the senior citizens home in silence. Here was a youth who was once scared to be alone in silence due to fear of his own monstrous thoughts. Now he relished and embraced the quietude. Silence was no longer scary for LaBoy, it was peaceful and comforting.

The youth rid himself of the demon energy that once encompassed him by forgiving himself. He was now the evicting Landlord of the painful thoughts that once plagued his mind. It was now time for the youth to move on and revitalize his creative spiritual force, a force that dwelled deep within.

Hawkinson looked the youth over as they walked. His aura no longer appeared murky and depleted. His step seemed lighter. He no longer walked as if he was an elephant carrying the weight of the world on his back. The mean scowl he once wore was replaced with a serene makeover. LaBoy had been resurrected.

*   *   *   *   *

When they entered the senior citizens home, LaBoy approached Sunflower. He asked if he could talk to her. After she agreed, Laboy apologized and asked her for forgiveness for the inhumane way he'd been demoralizing, objectifying and sexualizing her and the other female staff. The sincerity of the apology completely took her by surprise. Sunflower accepted the youth's apology and forgave him as she had already done when he was taken off the ban to all female staff. LaBoy thanked her before joining his peers. The apology was much more sincere than before.

"Okay, what in the hell just happened Hawk? Did I just step into the twilight zone or some sort of stargate worm hole?" Sunflower asked as she approached her colleague. "Did you prompt youth LaBoy to come up with that awesome apology?"

"I had nothing to do with it. It was all his doing."

Sunflower and Hawkinson observed closely as LaBoy approached the nurse of the deceased woman. He confessed to her his connection to her late aunt. She told him that her great aunt had already revealed his identity to her last Sunday evening. She smiled deeply and touched his shoulder thanking him for the courage he displayed and wished him well during his life journey.

*   *   *   *   *

It was the following Sunday, Fathers Day. For the first time in Hawkinson's eleven cycle tour at Lake Apache the annual Family Day cookout was scheduled the same day as Father's Day. The youth were allowed to invite up to four family members or supportive people in their lives for Family Day. Hawkinson, Minnis and the other male staff prepared for the celebration. Minnis sparked up the grill early that morning. He had a few of the youth assist him with the preparations. Hawkinson set up the games.

Family Day was an open house and celebration that the staff and youth put together every cycle. The day was all about reconciliation, recovery and reunification. It was no surprise that a great deal of family members were not invested. That's why a great deal of the youth were in the current position they were in; lack of support. There were no excuses for some of the families that claimed they didn't have transportation. Lake Apache provided transportation to and from the train and bus stations.

The morning would began with the youth paying tribute to the male staff on unit eight as well as inspirational father figures in their lives. After the tribute, the youth would visit with family members. After the visit came the best part of the day for most of the youth and their families— the cookout.

That morning as Hawkinson prepared to lead the Father Figure tribute held outdoors underneath the sun, the Lake Apache vehicles carrying family members began rolling in. The families were seated in the bleachers across from the track. Hawkinson led the ceremony. Each youth approached the podium one at a time as they discussed their definition of a father figure.

Youth Joby Kiddwell stood at the podium and paid tribute to a male employee from the Audi Home on the west side of Chicago who was visiting that day as his father figure. He chose him because he always looked out for him while he was serving time. The employee protected him from the older kids at the home. He fed the youth extra food when he was hungry and most importantly, he listened to the youth as well as offered him support.

Another youth from a small town chose to identify a firefighter who was visiting as his father figure. The fireman enrolled the youth in a volunteer program and taught him the ropes of becoming a great firefighter. The most important attribute the youth identified about the firefighter is that he spent time with him.

Another youth chose his uncle as a father figure. The uncle was a successful business man with a flourishing business. He allowed the youth to work at his establishment before he got into trouble with the law. He never turned his back on the youth and agreed to allow him to return to his establishment once he finished treatment.

Each young man approached the podium and shared their thoughts and feelings on father figures. Youth Averson, Franklin, Braylon Nicholson, Brennen, Sanchez and Geronimo named Minnis, Hawkinson and the other male staff as father figures. They were the men that educated them and spent countless hours molding and prepping them for success over the past ten months. The tribute turned out to be a grand event.

When the speeches were over, the family meet and greet hour began. Many of the youth were anxious to introduce their family members to Hawkinson, Sunflower, Minnis and the many other staff who were on site for the glorious event. LaBoy approached Hawkinson and Sunflower with his father by his side.

LaBoy Sr. extended his hand towards Hawkinson. While studying his eyes he firmly shook the calloused hand of the man he imagined to look much different in person. LaBoy Sr. then shifted his wolfish gaze to Maya Sunflower.

"Damn Jr, I see why you couldn't get no work done when you first got here," he said to his son as he looked Sunflower up and down in a deviant lustful manner. From his peripheral, Hawkinson could see Sunflower's nostrils flare and claws extend. He wisely stepped in while saying a silent prayer for LaBoy Sr. LaBoy Jr. looked away and lowered his head in shame.

"Ms. Sunflower, I think they may be needing your assistance over at the family Bingo tent," Hawkinson said trying to guide her away before she transformed into a fire breathing dragon, but it was too late. As professional as she could be, Sunflower released her wrath.

"You know sir, it's really too bad you have to model this type of behavior in front of your son. He deserves better, but now I understand why he once had to be put on ban to all female staff… he was just being a product of his environment. You have a good day now. Nice hat," she said walking away popping her knuckles.

"She's kind of feisty. I like that," LaBoy Sr. said as he chuckled loudly. He was an older man who was oddly dressed. The Berenstein Bears fishing hat that he wore was flipped up in the front. The twenty year old Members Only jacket he squeezed into hosted a pack of black and mild cigars in the upper pocket. The Steve Erkle suspenders had his pants hiked up close to his chest and the imitation snakeskin loafers appeared to be shedding their skin.

"Jr., go on over there and tell one of those women to fix me a plate of that bar-b-que before it's all gone," LaBoy Sr. told his son. LaBoy Jr. looked at Hawkinson with an uh-oh face.

"Boy, didn't you hear what I said. Now get over there and do as I say," he said in a degrading tone.

"Go on and get yourself something to eat son and let me talk to your father," Hawkinson said in a humble tone. LaBoy Jr. walked away with his head down.

LaBoy Sr. attempted to stare Hawkinson down for interfering and going against his command. The stare tactic was one that never intimidated Hawkinson. He always looked at the situation as an opportunity to learn more about a person. The eye gazing veteran looked directly in LaBoy Sr.'s eyes and read his soul in a matter of seconds.

From their interaction, Hawkinson could tell LaBoy Sr. was a bitter individual who was controlled, dominated and never loved as a child. As he grew physically, the little man internally stopped growing. The older physical LaBoy Sr. was now under the strict guidance and supervision of the little man controlling him from inside, the little man who lacked love for himself, his son and especially women.

LaBoy Sr. attacked Hawkinson with verbal daggers. He scoffed that he and the academy were making his son soft. Out of ignorance, he told Hawkinson his son would have been better off in jail than coming there learning some pompous, ass kissing way of living.

Hawkinson realized LaBoy Sr. spoke from fear. Fear that his son might in some way, make a better life for himself than he did. Hawkinson allowed him to speak without interfering. When all his ammo was gone, LaBoy Sr. stood before Hawkinson huffing and puffing out of breath. Hawkinson repeated what LaBoy Sr. said to him. It confirmed that he was listening. This was a therapeutic tool that Hawkinson used with the youth that proved to be very effective.

He now asked LaBoy Sr., for his undivided attention. The hostile bitter man folded his arms and looked away. The crossed arms, clenched teeth and heavy breathing were all signs that he was on the defense. Hawkinson lowered his voice in a clear but direct tone as he spoke his peace.

He shared with LaBoy Sr. the major accomplishments his son achieved since attending Lake Apache. He spoke about the elderly woman his son robbed while causing her to fall and break her hip. LaBoy Sr. continued to look away from Hawkinson. He told him while his son was doing volunteer work at a local nursing home he came face to face with the woman, but she passed away before he got a chance to go back the following week and apologize.

Hawkinson asked LaBoy Sr. to put himself in the position of the elderly woman who was robbed and asked what he would do if he had to sit down face to face with the assailant that attacked him? Only then did LaBoy Sr.

face Hawkinson and give him his undivided attention. For some reason, man always seems to respond when his safety has been threatened. LaBoy Sr. was no different.

After Hawkinson finished talking to him about all the wonderful things his son had accomplished, LaBoy Sr. in his own distorted, round about way, attempted to be a little less abrasive and more appreciative towards Hawkinson and the other Lake Apache staff.

Chapter 23

Loving Deeds for the Children:
A Man Called Hawk

(The power of giving)

After having the conversation with Hawkinson about his son's accomplishments, LaBoy Sr. confirmed that he would attend family therapy sessions for the next six weeks to support LaBoy Jr. Hawkinson developed the feeling that LaBoy Sr. was more than interested in supporting his son, he was interested in learning for himself, which was more than okay. In the short amount of time he spent with Hawkinson, LaBoy Sr. developed a great deal of respect for the man he had all but cursed. He shook Hawkinson's hand before walking away and allowing his nose to lead him over to the food tent.

LaBoy Jr. approached Hawkinson with a grim look on his face. He asked the calm reserved Hawkinson what he said to his father, because his father never shook hands with anyone. Hawkinson told the youth that his father was just confirming that he was looking forward to the family therapy sessions. LaBoy Jr. used his hand to cover up the smile that stretched across his face. Hawkinson told the youth it was okay to be excited as he patted him on the shoulder before walking away to socialize.

"Mr. Hawkinson," LaBoy Jr. called out.

"Yes sir," Hawkinson said turning to face the youth.

"Thank you for being the father figure I wish my dad could have been."

"You're welcome," he said smiling at the youth before walking away with his usual confident swagger. Hawkinson walked around socializing with the many guests. An aunt of one of the youth who had a great admiration for Minnis' grilled ribs attempted to get her nephew to play matchmaker for her with Hawkinson. The humble servant was flattered but declined the offer as he strolled off in pursuit of more conversation.

*   *   *   *   *

Graduation was just a month away. Things were becoming quite intense. Hawkinson was meeting with the youth for therapy sessions as well as meeting with some of the families after their session with the family therapist. After two family therapy sessions, LaBoy Sr. was still abrasive and obnoxious as ever but he was invested. Being invested meant he cared and that was good enough for Hawkinson.

*   *   *   *   *

Hawkinson met with youth Brennen for a session. The youth brought up his very first encounter with him when they were walking over to the dining hall. The youth admitted how intimidated he was that day, but how grateful he was later that Hawkinson showed care and concern by challenging and correcting his behavior. Hawkinson reminisced as he chuckled at the thought of Brennen making up the story of honey and celery.

After taking Hawkinson on a tour through his memory museum, Brennen expressed that he was struggling with multiple issues. One of the main issues was returning to his family in his home state of Kentucky. The youth was worried that despite his changes, everything and everybody else would be the same, including his alcoholic mother. He worried that the temptation of drugs and alcohol would cause him to be like his mother and his imprisoned father. The supportive counselor listened to the youth in detail before offering minimum suggestions. After accepting Hawkinson's suggestions, Brennen asked a question.

"Don't you ever worry about failing?"

"Failing is an illusion of the mind. Your level of success solely depends on your thoughts. If you see yourself as a failure, you will fail. If you see yourself as a shining superstar, you will succeed and shine," Hawkinson said as he pressed the button to the cd player on his desk. The song *Superstar* by Lupe Fiasco began to play. Brennen's blue eyes lit up as he smiled deeply and bobbed his head to the sound of the music while singing the opening lyrics. Hawkinson smiled as the youth rocked it out.

When the song ended, Hawkinson asked the youth how he felt. With wide eyes and an adrenaline rush, he responded with, "great!" Hawkinson commended him for having a good session and told him he would see him later. Youth Brennen continued singing the lyrics to the song as he stood and approached the door. When he reached the door he turned around to face Hawkinson.

"Excuse me Mr. Hawkinson?"

"Yes sir," he said looking up.

"I know we look nothing alike and we come from two different worlds, but thank you for being a supportive father figure to me," the thin youth said with a straight face.

"You're welcome. It's all about the deeds youth Brennen," Hawkinson said.

"Not just any deeds Mr. Hawkinson, but loving deeds for us children," the youth said before leaving the office. Hawkinson was touched by the youth's sincerity. Brennen was ice cold when he first arrived at Lake Apache. It was a pleasure for Hawkinson to see the youth warm up and start investing in his life.

*   *   *   *   *

Hawkinson met with the seven youth for the relaxation meditation group. Many of them were quite comfortable and advanced in the group by now. In fact, they were so advanced they didn't need Hawkinson to visually guide them anymore. The youth created their own place of peace during the meditation.

As the music played, Hawkinson observed the physical changes of the youth who once displayed extreme anger problems. The hard lines and frowns in their faces melted away. Their faces became alive and lit up with spiritual force.

The youth were calm and relaxed as their heads and shoulders slumped. Their chins rested on their chest. It was a sure sign that they were totally relaxed and unwound. Meditation was like medication for many of them. When Hawkinson brought them back from their imaginative place of peace, many didn't want to return. The mansions in their minds were the safest places they'd ever been. It made sense to not want to return.

After processing their experiences, the youth exited the group very relaxed and stress free. Again, the peers outside of the group took notice of the calmness their peers displayed as they stared unbelievably. The majority of those youth wanted to immediately sign up to join the group. It was a major compliment for the man called Hawk who provided loving deeds for the children.

*   *   *   *   *

It'd been some time since Hawkinson met with Thadius Powers for an individual session. After the youth was put on ban to Sunflower for therapeutic reasons, he flat out refused to meet with Hawkinson or any of the other therapists. He shut down which left him at a treatment stand still. The troubled youth sat across from Hawkinson with a bizarre look in his eyes. Deeply, he still blamed the senior counselor for messing up his distorted relationship with Sunflower.

Hawkinson sat quietly until the youth was ready to process. The silence didn't seem to bother the socially inadequate misfit who had spent several days at a time in confinement when he was in corrections. When Hawkinson would write something in his notes the youth would grow paranoid and attempted to catch a glimpse of what was on the paper. When he would look up from his notes, the youth would look away. Curiosity was starting to get the best of Powers. He asked Hawkinson what was he writing. He responded by informing him he was taking notes on his session.

"But I haven't said anything," Powers said.

"Exactly," Hawkinson said still writing.

"I was told in order to graduate I had to attend these shitty individual sessions."

"You do."

"Well I'm fricking here."

"But you're not actively participating."

"Goddamn it man, what do you fricking want me to say?" he asked in a frustrated tone popping up on the edge of his chair in an aggressive manner.

"Whatever comes to heart and mind," Hawkinson responded looking the youth square in the eye. The aggravated youth stomped his foot as he slammed back in his chair with such force, nearly knocking himself over. He began grunting and twisting in his chair trying to control the developing rage within. Hawkinson stopped writing and sat his pen down, touched his fingers together and slightly leaned forward on the edge of his chair.

Powers began releasing animalistic type sounds and grunts as tears streamed down his face. Hawkinson assured the youth he was there, ready to listen and support whenever he was ready to release. The disturbed behaviors went on for the next several minutes before Powers calmed down and spoke.

He told Hawkinson repeatedly how much he hated himself for allowing others to treat him like crap all his life. Not only did he hate himself, he hated his mother for not being there for him, and he hated the people who were there. Powers was a system baby from birth. His mother was a cocaine addict. Before she gave birth to Thadius, his four other brother and sisters were removed from the home by the Department of Children & Family Services (DCFS). Powers expressed that he became a ward of the state barely out of the womb.

It was evident to Hawkinson that the youth was a drug baby. His distorted features and extreme lack of impulse control proved to be self-evident. The youth went on to tell Hawkinson that his first memory ever was watching one of his foster mother's boyfriends ram her head through a glass window. He was no older than three to four years of age. He remembered crying and no one attending to him in the midst of the chaos. The boyfriend would beat on her and she in return would beat on the children. The youth expressed that many times, he would be flung across the room or tossed into a chair because of his hyperactivity. The only way the foster mother felt she could control the children was the way her boyfriend controlled her, through physical aggression. The youth stared off into space as he ventured off into the next part of his life.

DCFS intervened again and placed him with another foster family. He stayed with this particular family until he was about eight. Powers expressed that the home was governed by a foster mom that dictated orders from the couch while watching a television that was her pride and joy. He said she ate tv dinners, read tv magazines and slept on the couch in front of her tv. The foster mother loved her t.v. so much that none of the seven children could touch or watch her television unless they watched what she was watching.

One day the house mysteriously caught on fire. One of the children tried to tell the foster mother but she was too busy lying on the couch watching tv. By the time the foster mom smelled the smoke it was too late. The flames spread throughout the house quickly. Fortunately everyone escaped unharmed, even the foster mother who never got off the couch except to use the restroom and go to the refrigerator.

"Everything in the house burned up, especially that goddamn tv," Powers said with a deviant smile as he relived the moment. He continued by telling Hawkinson that the foster mother neglected him, which according to him was worse than any physical abuse he ever endured. Powers was happy that the foster mother lost her tv, but he was sad that he and all the other children had to split up and go to other foster homes.

"Did you start the fire and burn up the tv?" Hawkinson asked Powers. The youth cleared his throat and chose not to answer. Hawkinson took the response as a yes. Powers continued by discussing the next family that took him in. He was placed in a foster home with a woman who had two sons and a daughter. He said at first everything was going along nicely. The boys treated him like a younger brother and the mother and daughter took him everywhere with them.

Shortly after his eleventh birthday, Powers expressed shamefully that certain things began to happen to him. He told Hawkinson he secretly began looking at the physical shape and form of his foster mom and sister.

"How'd it make you feel?" Hawkinson asked.

"Nervous and scared, but excited at the same time," the youth said as he shyly looked away. Hawkinson encouraged him to continue. The youth expressed that he developed a deep interest in his foster sister. He began secretly reading her diary and going through her dresser drawers. He admitted that he became obsessed. When she would have sleepovers, she would let him be the gopher to bring snacks and treats to her friends. Powers went on to express that he became so fixated on his foster sister that he began having dreams about her.

"What kind of dreams?" Hawkinson asked. Powers began butterflying his legs rapidly as he thought of a way to tell Hawkinson about the dreams.

"Wet dreams," the youth said in a subtle tone.

"Oh, you mean nocturnal emissions, totally normal for most males at that age," Hawkinson said in a non-chalant tone of voice. He asked the youth what attracted him to the foster sister. Powers responded by admitting she was genuinely nice to him, just like Miss Sunflower. Powers thought back to all the different times Sunflower paid him the slightest attention and showed him a little care and concern, which was something she did with all the youth when they first arrived to the academy. The youth spent weeks creating fantasies and distorting her meekness for weakness and her kindness for blindness.

Powers continued by sharing that one day when his foster sister and mother were away, he entered the sister's bedroom as he did before and began snooping around. He dug around in one of her drawers until he found her diary. He sat on her bed and began reading her latest private thoughts.

The oldest of the two foster brothers entered the room and caught him reading the diary. He laughed and told Powers he was so busted. He then began teasing that he was going to tell his sister that he was reading her diary and snooping around in her underwear drawer. As the brother turned to leave, his sister was standing in the doorway.

Powers spoke about the look on her face. It was a look of violation. She charged and cursed him as she threw anything she could get her hands on at him. Powers ran out of the house and hid. Later that evening when he returned to the house the entire family along with a DCFS worker were sitting at the kitchen table. From the look on their faces, he knew it wasn't good. He was told to pack up his things. The mother called him a pervert and told him she no longer wanted him under her roof with her daughter.

Powers said he remembered feeling so hurt and embarrassed that he couldn't even look at the mother or the daughter. While packing his things he took on the role of a victim. He blamed the family for him having to leave. Out of revenge, he stole his foster brother's authentic vintage baseball card collection. He smeared lipstick and makeup all over his foster mother's dresses and shoes. He then went into his foster sister's room, took her favorite stuffed animal and stuffed it down the rear of his pants and released a bowel movement. He sat the stuffed animal in the middle of her bed before grabbing his bags and leaving the house with the state worker. Later he remembered feeling disgusted with himself for what he did.

"Where did you learn the behavior of defecating onto stuffed animals?" Hawkinson asked the youth. Powers paused, as his eyes grew cold and distant. It was clear to Hawkinson the youth was reliving the trauma.

"I learned it from my first foster mom's boyfriend. She bought me a stuffed animal for my seventh birthday party. He crashed the party drunk as a bama skunk. She told him to leave because he was ruining my party. He looked at me, grabbed my stuffed animal and shoved me to the floor before pulling down his pants and wiping his ass with it. He then held me down and smeared it in my face. I didn't know what embarrassed and belittled meant at that time, but I sure know what it felt like." Hawkinson asked Powers to continue.

The youth said after leaving the foster family home he was taken to an emergency shelter while waiting for the approval of another foster family to take him in. While staying at the shelter the police arrived looking for him. He was taken to the jail for criminal damage to property. The family wanted to press charges. He told Hawkinson the arresting officer was the boyfriend of the foster mother. Out of revenge, he placed the youth in a cell with adult male offenders.

Powers grew quiet as tears leaked from his wide eyes. He told Hawkinson the men had their way with him over and over again. The message from the arresting officer was that he would never take a crap on anyone else's possessions. Powers was released the next day to a state worker. The youth said he never told a soul about the stuffed animal or jail experience until now. He told Hawkinson instead of the incident being a deterent for him, he grew more hateful and resentful to every authority figure that he came across. Powers became his own superhero and villan, and as sick as it sounds the movement of his bowels became his power. As superman had x-ray vision and spiderman had web shooters, Thadius Powers had his excrement. It became his weapon of choice. He defecated all over the town leaving fecal matter on the doorsteps of those he deemed an enemy. That along with other heinous crimes landed the youth in the Department of Corrections.

"Is that how the story goes?" Hawkinson asked.

"Yes sir, that's how the story goes," the youth said with a superficial grin. As they sat in silence, the grin was soon replaced by an upside down smile. Powers began tearing up.

Hawkinson watched the outer casing break away and fall freely from the youth. His fragile insides were exposed for the first time. Hawkinson no longer saw an eighteen year old beastly acting youth offender sitting before him. Therapeutically, he saw a little boy who had conformed to his early childhood environment.

Powers removed himself from the chair and lay on the rug in Hawkinson's office. He curled up in the fetal position and cradled himself as he rocked back and forth. The youth cried as if he was a baby longing for his mother's loving touch. The pain within that bellowed out was so horrifying it brought a few of Hawkinson's colleagues including Sunflower running to the door. Hawkinson held up a hand halting them.

Sunflower curiously peered over the desk to see Powers curled up on the floor. She looked at Hawkinson and shrugged her shoulders. He signaled to her and his other colleagues that everything was fine. They backed out of the doorway and left Hawkinson alone with the healing youth.

One of the main things Hawkinson loved about the team he was blessed to be a part of was their care, concern and support. They looked out for one another. Sure, they had their disagreements and other petty issues but they always kept one another safe.

Chapter 24
Graduation
(The Rites of Passage)

The cycle was winding down. It was almost graduation. Youth scurried around to get the last of their treatment assignments completed. The last two volunteer groups completed their volunteer services in the community. LaBoy Sr. and other parents were showing up weekly for family services. Although he had attended just four family sessions, Hawkinson could see a difference in LaBoy Sr.'s attitude. It wasn't a major change, but it was still a change. He was even able to hold a respectful conversation with Sunflower and the other female staff without objectifying and projecting his insecurity issues onto them.

*   *   *   *   *

Hawkinson sat at his desk writing notes for an evening group before the youth returned from school. He heard extreme laughter and celebrating out near the staff's lounge. He stood and exited the office.

"Wow Hawk, unbelievable," a male colleague said to him as he walked by. Hawkinson looked at him suspiciously. The colleague looked over his shoulder and chuckled as he disappeared around the corner. Hawkinson approached the lounge door and entered. A group of his peers were gathered around the news bulletin board. The group spotted Hawkinson making his way toward them. The laughter subsided as everyone evacuated the area like roaches exposed to light. They snickered as they walked away. Sunflower was standing at the bulletin board smiling with her arms folded as Hawkinson approached the board. The results from the physical performance test were posted.

"Read 'em and weep Hawkster," Sunflower said as she patted her trusty co-worker on the back before walking away. Hawkinson read the results of the physical performance test. He used his finger to guide him down the alphabetically arranged list. When he got to the H's he spotted his name and smiled after he read his score. He then searched downward towards the S's. He read Sunflower's score. Immediately the smile that once brightened his face disappeared and was replaced by a look of disbelief.

Sunflower called his name. As soon as he turned to face her, she snapped his photo with the look of disbelief still tattooed on his face. The entire lounge of colleagues went into an uproar. Hawkinson was at a loss for words for the first time in his career.

Sunflower outscored him by seven points during the final performance test of the cycle. It was the first time in the seven cycles of working together that she performed better than her overly competitive colleague. Sunflower made sure she basked in the glory and rubbed it in his face.

Although Hawkinson always set the bar high for himself and was more driven than a high performance Nascar, he was a good sport about finishing second behind Sunflower. He approached and gave her a high five. The fact that she outperformed him was a true testament to her powerful determination and stick-to-it-ive-ness.

Hawkinson walked back to his office not feeling defeated, but proud of Sunflower for her accomplishment. He reminisced back to her first cycle after the final physical performance test, which he won by a landslide. Sunflower vowed to Hawkinson that one day she was going to score higher than him. He told her the day he walked with a walker and carried around an oxygen tank would be the day she out performed him.

When Hawkinson entered his office, he bellied over and laughed hysterically. He laughed until tears streamed from his eyes. Sitting next to his desk was a walker and an oxygen tank. Sitting on the desk was a small basket of healing ointments for joints and cramps. Attached to the basket was a card. Still laughing from the surprise, Hawkinson opened the card and began reading:

Hey Hawk,

I know you're probably still crying your eyes out and licking your wounds while you're reading this card, but don't take it personally, just take it in as you always say. As a matter of fact, you have quite a few sayings like, *The Sun is always shining even when the skies are gray. B.E.L.I.E.V.E.-- The Best Ever Living Individual Evolving Very Excellently*, and one of my favorites of all times, *It is what it is*. So you see Hawk, I didn't take it personally when your competitive, overachieving drive dusted me twice a year for the past seven years. And you're right, the sun is always shining, even when the skies are gray. Well guess what? Today the sun is shining on me and according to the results of the physical performance test, the gray skies are directly above your head. And as far as being the best ever living individual evolving very excellently…thanks to you I am every bit of that as well. Thank you Horus Orion Hawkinson for being a great colleague, mentor, support, shoulder to lean on and most importantly… the other half of this dynamic duo.

Always and 4 ever, Maya Sunflower

Hawkinson closed the card and and placed it in the top drawer of the desk. He took another look at the walker and oygen tank before bellowing out another laughing spell. Sunflower had quite the humorous imagination.

*   *   *   *   *

Later that day, Hawkinson met with youth Roosevelt Franklin for an individual session. Despite the fears he was struggling with concerning life after Lake Apache, he was making great improvements. Although he had concerns about the uncertainty of his future in regards to locating his mother and biological family, the youth ran down a list of goals he'd been diligently working on to make sure he stayed focused. When the session came to an end, Roosevelt stood and approached the door. He turned around slowly with a perplexed look.

"Excuse me Mr. Hawkinson, but what's the walker and oxygen tank for?"

"Oh, that's just something I have to return to… you know ugh… the place where it came from," he said clearing his throat and stroking the center of his forehead with his index finger.

"I thought it may have been for you. Word on the streets is Ms. Sunflower dusted you pretty bad in the staff physical performance test. I don't know Mr.

Hawkinson, I think you may be at the top of the hill headed down really fast," the youth said as he exited the office shaking his head.

"It was only by seven points," Hawkinson called out.

*   *   *   *   *

As the date of the graduation neared, Hawkinson met individually with more of the youth. Tempers were escalating and anxiety was at an all time high. Some were starting to mentally check out and eliminate treatment from their vocabulary just as others did in the past. The tough Tony and Billy Bad Ass attitudes returned to the unit. Hawkinson clearly understood what was taking place. Many of the youth were having anxiety about leaving, which was completely understandable. After all, they spent the past eleven months in a safe structured environment with multiple support systems while healing themselves. Now they were headed back to society where no one cared about them or their issues. There would be no more processing feelings with a counselor or therapist whenever a problem arised. The youth learned early in life that the world is a very cold and frigid place, a place where it was almost time to return.

Hawkinson didn't expect the youth to change their lives in eleven months under the treatment umbrella. It was going to take more than that amount of time to penetrate through the concrete layers that tombed the little child within. Many were set up with an after care treatment plan. The plan was for the youth to receive outpatient counseling for six months while staying connected with a follow-up therapy team at Lake Apache.

*   *   *   *   *

While meeting with Joby the eve before graduation, Hawkinson heard loud swearing and threats near the dorms. Before he could make it to the door of his office, he heard ironing boards crashing to the floor and the squeaky sound that shoes make when there's a tussle going on.

When he and Joby reached the milieu, Sunflower and a male staff had Averson hemmed up in a corner. Minnis and two other staff had Powers in a therapeutic treatment hold while the other youth were being guided away from the area. The raging Averson struggled greatly to get at Powers. From the looks of it, one of the youth was ironing his clothes for the graduation while the other tried to take over. Powers was guided away to another area.

Hawkinson had Joby go with the others. He approached Sunflower and the male staff to assist with calming Averson down. Hawkinson stood before the youth and placed a hand on his shoulder. At a turtle's pace, Averson began to slow his struggle and breathing. Hawkinson signaled for the male staff to release his hold. The staff followed the signal. When Averson calmed down completely, he signaled for Sunflower to let him go. She released her hold and stepped aside. Hawkinson stood face to face with Averson with his hand still resting on his shoulder. The mood was now calm in the milieu. All the excitement and intense energy was flushed out. Hawkinson focused on the silence.

Ten minutes into the silence, he released his hand from Averson's shoulder before asking him to go stand at the exit door. The youth followed the directive as asked. Hawkinson then asked Sunflower to have Minnis and the other two staff bring Powers to the exit door. When Powers arrived, Hawkinson motioned for the youth to stand at the door as well. Minnis and two other staff stood between the two youth. Hawkinson and Sunflower gathered the rest of the youth and lined them up before marching them all out to the lake.

*   *   *   *   *

After all the youth were standing around the lake, Hawkinson commanded them to have a seat. It was near nightfall, the twilight hour. A couple of the counselors set up lanterns around the outside of the group. Hawkinson shared the story of Lake Apache with the youth. The theme of the story was about embracing courage while standing in the presence of fear. It was a powerful inspiring story Hawkinson shared with all the youth from the past.

He began the story with, *"Many moons ago a young fearless warrior escaped a dreaded battle that took place in the Southwestern states. The warrior traveled and settled in the midwest. He settled in a small Illinois town called Cahokia. There he banded together with other young warriors. When the battle spread from the southwest to the Midwest, wiping out other tribes including the Cahokia tribe along the way, the group of banded warriors headed further east until they settled on the very soil I'm standing on."*

Hawkinson had all the youths' undivided attention as he continued to tell the story. *"The warriors were followed to the lake by a brigade of outlaws. An ensuing battle broke out around the lake. The young warrior and his comrades were greatly outnumbered but they fought relentlessly. With nowhere to run and his back to the lake, the young warrior intelligently used the power of the water spirit from the lake as an ally. He chanted a mantra that turned the water from the lake into a great mist. The young warriors lured the attackers close to the lake. Because the outlaws were unfamiliar with the area, when they attacked, they fell off the ridge into the lake. The lake and the mist swallowed up the entire brigade of outlaws except for one. The one outlaw escaped. He told other outlaws and bandits that the small band of warriors defeated his entire brigade near a haunted lake and if they valued their lives, they should never encounter the warriors that resided near the lake."*

Hawkinson noticed the youth studying the peaceful serene lake. *"After the battle the young fearless warrior named the lake, Lake Apache after his tribal name. The young warrior and his band of warriors swore on an oath that they would protect and honor the lake and the land that surrounded it. They would one day have children and their children would carry on the oath and the legacy of Lake Apache."* By this time, the late evening sky transformed from orange and blue to black. Stars danced magically above on the night's canvas.

"Many many moons later when the young warrior's hair was no longer black as coal but had turned white as snow, he passed on and returned to the gates in the sky leaving a legacy behind. The retired warrior according to the legend returned to the heavens on a solar boat that ascended from the sky and landed on Lake Apache. The boat carried the warrior home across the sky. The boat then passed through the star gates in the sky. After the boat passed through the gates, a star cluster took on the form of a hawk headed warrior in the sky now known as Orion's belt. The warrior held a spear in one hand and a shield in the other." Hawkinson then pointed upwards and outwards to the Orion constellation in the southeastern part of the sky. He pointed out the three stars around the warrior's belt and the spear and shield in each hand.

The youth and all the staff sat in silence looking up at the night sky. Whatever worries and fears the many youth had before coming out to the lake were now gone. Hawkinson had captured them all with the legendary story.

He asked the youth to give their worries and fears to the warrior in the sky. He walked around and handed each youth a helium filled balloon before asking them to imaginatively place each worry and fear inside the ballon. When they were ready, he instructed the youth to release the balloons to the sky.

Each youth released his balloon to the sky. The lanterns lit up the balloons as they soared high into the night sky. When the last balloon disappeared out of sight, Hawkinson asked the youth to create a circle around him and lock arms. The youth created a circle as instructed and locked arms.

He told the youth in order to become warriors they had to pass the final test. The final test was to band together as one and to never let anyone tear them apart or break into their circle. His objective was to find the weakest link by trying to break through their link. Hawkinson approached Geronimo who was locked arms with Braylon and another youth. He began to push his way through the youth. They held strong. Hawkinson pushed harder, but the youth stayed linked together. He backed off as he began to bead up with perspiration. Sweat dripped from the top of his head down his face.

"One of you will break the link and let me out of this circle! I can feel it! You're not warriors yet so that means somewhere in this chain there is a weak link," he said looking around the circle. Hawkinson was a master at studying body language. He spotted two peers who were not appropriately locked.

"Are you going to let me break down your chain tonight?"

"No sir!" the youth shouted from the depths of their souls.

"I can't hear you!" he shouted out.

"Nooooo! Sirrrrr!" the youth said getting pumped as they tightened the chain. Hawkinson quickly approached the two youth with the weak hold.

"Here he comes! Lock it down! Lock at the hips!" Geronimo called out as he noticed the weak hold by his peers. Just before Hawkinson reached the two youth, they locked at the hip and beared down as he tried to push through for seconds at a time. Unsuccessful, Hawkinson backed off.

"Somebody's going to let me break through tonight! I can feel it!" he said in a deepened voice as he went to youth after youth trying to break through the chain. By now he was saturated in sweat and so were most of the youth.

"As of now I represent all the fear, worry, pain and suffering any of you have ever endured. I am the enemy that has kept you from succeeding! If I break you down, I win! Are you going to let me break you down!"

"Nooooo Sirrrrr!" the youth screamed and shouted. Hawkinson spotted what may have been the weakest link in the chain. Averson and Powers were linked together. He knew the two hadn't resolved their petty differences from earlier. Averson locked eyes with Hawkinson. Hawkinson began smiling. Averson looked at Powers who was trembling from exhaustion and barely hanging on. Hawkinson charged the two youth at full speed.

"Here he comes man! Lock it down man! Lock it down!" Averson screamed out to Powers. As Hawkinson approached and attempted to push his way through, Powers began grunting and screaming as he held onto Averson with everything he had. Together, both of the youth pushed forward. Hawkinson stumbled backwards. He charged in again and tried to break through. This time he could feel the link loosening. He could feel Powers giving in as he pushed and pushed. Geronimo screamed out and told his peers to have no fear and believe in the power of love, something Hawkinson had been teaching them since day one. Geronimo then began chanting Love!

"Love! Love! Love!" he continued until all of his peers joined in and began chanting as well. The force of the chant was too powerful and overwhelming for Hawkinson. He retreated to the middle of the circle out of breath. He reached into his back pocket and pulled out a cloth towel. He wiped his head and face while observing the youth. All was sound. He lowered the white towel along his side. The youth locked down even tighter as they stopped chanting and stared him down. Hawkinson smiled widely before waving the towel into the air surrendering. The youth broke loose from the chain cheering and celebrating by hugging and high fiving one another. Averson and Geronimo lifted Powers onto their shoulders and paraded him around with their peers following behind. Hawkinson was proud of the no longer youth, but band of warriors as he watched them parade around.

"That's two defeats in one week. You're making it a pretty bad habit Hawk," Sunflower said smiling as she approached her colleague with a cool bottle of water.

In all the previous cycles, Hawkinson always found a weak link and broke through the chains, but not that night. The youth of this cycle had something the other youth of the past didn't have. They had love and a bond. They believed in the power of love that bonded them together. After the youth celebrated, Hawkinson and his colleagues pulled them all together.

He told them that night they were no longer youth of Lake Apache Academy. They were warriors of a new light, a new truth and a new spiritual resurrection. They showed resilience and determination by completing the rite of passage. The youth took the practical blueprint application that Hawkinson and his colleagues provided and they applied it. That blueprint application was love—loving deeds for the children. Hawkinson told the youth on the count of three he was going to ask who are we and they were to respond by screaming warriors at the top of their voices.

"1...2...3...Who are we?" Hawkinson asked.

"Warriors!"

"Who are we?" he asked again.

"Warriors!"

"I... can't... hear you! You sound like one little knat at a Sunday afternoon picnic! Who are we?" he asked as loud as he could.

"Warrrriorrrrs!!!!!" the youth shouted with everything they had as the reverberating sound of their voices carried off and faded into the blackness of night.

*   *   *   *   *

The next morning all the youth were dressed neatly and lined up in a row in the parking lot, ready to march over to the complex for the graduation ceremony. The early morning July sun illuminated them all. Geronimo stood before his peers carrying the Warriors flag. Behind him were Averson, Brennen and Franklin carrying flags that represented the three colors of the phase system.

Hawkinson and his colleagues looked the youth over. Hygiene was right, haircuts were tight and smiles were bright. Hawkinson was proud of every youth that stood before him. Never in the history of Lake Apache had all the youth who entered the same cycle at the same time graduated together. Joby was the only holdover from the past cycle and even he was graduating.

The youth arrived to the complex and sat down on the unit eight side. There were over two hundred graduates combined from the eight units. It was exciting times for the youth. Most had never accomplished anything in their lives. Now they were about to walk across a stage and receive an honorary certificate and plaque for their dedication to eleven months of cognitive based treatment.

*   *   *   *   *

When the graduation was over that early afternoon, the unit eight warriors returned to the unit for a small ceremony and celebration. During the celebration, the youth honored the staff with cards and gifts they made from their creative imaginations.

Braylon was the first of his peers to approach Hawkinson with a gift. He handed him a symbol of eternal life crafted from wood. He also painted Hawkinson a portrait of a warrior with angel wings and a hawk head.

Geronimo was the next of his peers to approach Hawkinson. The graduated warrior first thanked him for all that he taught him and for being a father figure, a rolemodel and spiritual teacher. The gift Geronimo handed Hawkinson was a decorated warrior's tomahawk with a coyote symbol cut into the ivory stone. He also made him a warrior's mask made from paper mache`. Hawkinson shook the youth's hand and thanked him from the core of his heart.

The next to bear a gift was Brennen. He thanked Hawkinson for being a father figure. He told the senior counselor he never met anyone that treated young people with so much respect and tough love. He told him he would never forget him for as long as he lived. He presented Hawkinson with a warriors mask made of clay that was baked in a kiln. It was an amazing craft of art. It resembled the shades of blue warriors mask hanging in his office.

The next youth to present was Roosevelt Franklin. He dedicated a collage of words and pictures to Hawkinson that he encased in glass. The collage was inscripted with all of the youths' ambitions, desires and dreams. The collage also displayed what he wanted to be professionally, important events in his life, favorite movie, favorite book, family members, food and his favorite hero, which was Hawkinson. The gift was genuine and it was created from the heart of a child turned warrior.

Hawkinson received many more gifts from the youth. The last one to approach was Averson. He was already starting to tear up. Unlike the other youth that shook Hawkinson's hand, Averson reached out and wrapped his arms around him. Hawkinson embraced the warrior and supported his time of emotional expression.

After allowing his emotions to flow freely, Averson stepped back and handed his role model a book. It was a book that the youth overheard Hawkinson discussing that he wanted to purchase. Hawkinson thanked Averson greatly.

"Everything that I ever wanted to say to you… I wrote it inside the front cover of this book," the somewhat bashful youth said. Hawkinson opened the book and began reading.

Mr. Hawkinson~

I hope you like the book. You are a great teacher with a great heart. You are a real man. You have taught me so much. Thank you for assisting me in my spiritual resurrection. I once felt dead, but I can now say I am truly living. I hope that you are able to achieve every goal you have set 4 yourself. The energy that you carry within is genuinely unbelievable. You do great things Mr. Hawkinson, and I know through the law of cause and effect great things will be returned to you. You have been a great friend and inspiring teacher to me, and that is a priceless gift that I would not trade for anything. No matter how wise a master may be there are always new things to learn, so keep climbing up "Jacobs Ladder!" Thank you for everything Mr. Hawkinson May the light of the eternal source always be with you.

Your Warrior brother 4 ever, Marley Averson!

Hawkinson closed the book and smiled.

"You have a bright future ahead of you youth Averson," Hawkinson said giving him a soulful handshake. "Don't ever hesitate to pick up the phone and call, I'll be here."

"I know you will Mr. Hawkinson, just like the sun that's always shining, even when the skies are gray."

*   *   *   *   *

The last of the young warriors left the campus shortly after 1400 hours. The cycle was finally over. Hawkinson had another notch on his belt of success as a Senior Therapeutic Youth Counselor. He and his peers had five weeks off before the next cycle began. Because there were no holdovers, no one had to stay over and work their summer break. One by one, the staff gathered their things and departed for their well deserved time off.

Hawkinson and Sunflower were the last two standing in the parking lot. They discussed what they were going to do for their break. Sunflower was going to fly out of the country to vacation, but not before going back home to Phoenix to visit her family. She invited Hawkinson to come out and visit the desert at the end of every cycle and every cycle he accepted the offer but the overly active go-getter never made time for the trip. She promised him if he came this summer, they would take a drive up to Sedona, a spiritual place he always wanted to visit.

For the first couple of weeks of his time off, Hawkinson was running a basketball camp and a youth work study program for teenagers in an underpriviledged area of the county. He promised Sunflower on his time off he would visit her native state.

"Okay Hawk, I have to go. I have a lot of highway before me. Before I blink my eyes, it'll be time to be right back for a new and exciting adventure. Thanks for all your support. This has been no doubt the most successful and interesting cycle we've had."

"So I guess that means you're coming back," he said eyeing the physical performance trophy Sunflower carried proudly.

"Of course I'll be back. What would you do without me, and I'm going to go out on a limb and say… you're not getting this trophy back. Next cycle I'm coming back new and improved, stronger, better and faster."

"Good, because I'm going to be stronger, better, faster and all that other stuff."

"Do you ever stop competing? Be good and stay out of trouble," she said hugging her co-worker.

"I can't make any promises, somehow trouble always seems to find me," he said hugging her in return. Sunflower loaded her car with personal items and gifts she received from the youth. She smiled deviantly and looked at Hawkinson's car suspiciously before getting into her car. As she sped off, Sunflower honked her horn and waved.

Hawkinson waved in return as he walked around to get into his car. He looked down at the front tire and noticed something yellow on it. It was a boot. Sunflower booted his car. Hawkinson looked up in the direction she drove off and attempted to call her name, but instead he couldn't do anything but laugh. He laughed hysterically until his sides hurt. Maya Sunflower had pranked him again.

A few minutes later, she returned to the parking lot with tears from laughter streaming down her face. Maya pulled up next to Hawkinson. He looked at her and shook his head.

"What? I couldn't resist," she said laughing it up even more. After the laughing spell ended, she told Hawkinson the tool to unlock the boot was in the storage shed next to unit eight's building.

"What do you want me to do with this thing once I get it off?" Hawkinson asked.

"I thought you could take it to basketball camp with you, so when the children cross you over and break your ankle, you'll already have a protective boot," she said chuckling.

"You're just full of humor today. Did one of the graduates buy you a joke book before they left?" Hawkinson asked as he mimicked Sunflower's laughter.

"Bye Hawk. Hope you have a good camp and I look forward to seeing you in a couple of weeks. Don't stand me up," Maya said before honking her horn and driving off.

As Hawkinson removed the boot from his tire a large shadow flew overhead and blocked out the sun. When he looked up at the clear skies, Hawkinson noticed a hawk circling above. It was carrying a sunflower in its mouth as it swooped down just inches above his head before soaring back up into the sky. He watched the hawk until it disappeared out of sight.

Hawkinson finished removing the boot. He put it away and studied his surroundings. The parking lot was empty. The campus itself seemed like a ghost town compared to early that morning. Everyone had departed except for the few holdovers and staff on other programs. Five more weeks and Hawkinson would be back at it again, ready for a new adventure, new challenges and new experiences.

No one outside the walls of Lake Apache could ever understand what Hawkinson and his colleagues endured on a daily basis. The professional men and women of Lake Apache made up brother and sisterhoods that offered their loving, Godly deeds for the children. They confided in one another, supported one another and looked to one another for strength. They were an alliance of superheroes that provided a practical blueprint application for the youth of the past and those to come in the future. That blueprint is love.

It was a Saturday afternoon, and Hawkinson had the rest of the day and Sunday before basketball camp began. He got into his car, started it up and opened the sunroof. The radiant energy from the star of life above spiraled down, energizing his aura. Hawkinson was happy loving life and in return, life was loving him back. He turned on the stereo. One of the greatest tunes of all time by the legendary Al Green, entitled *Love and Happiness* flowed from the speakers and out the sunroof, as a man called Hawk drove away for some fun under the sun.

Acknowledgments

I would like to first give thanks to the Prime Creator, the many positive forces of the universe and the Christ consciousness that freely flowed through me while working diligently on this novel. I would also like to thank the hundreds of children I've coached, counseled and mentored for allowing me to provide you with loving deeds. You all have challenged me beyond heights and taken me on a journey I couldn't have imagined in my wildest dreams. Without any of you, this novel would not and could not be possible. I am universally grateful to you all.

To Linda Ragsdale and the wonderful Ladies of Beverly Book Club, thank you for reading my previous novel, *Dream Weaver the Indigo* and having me as a guest at your January 2008 book club gathering. Your hospitality and warmth was appreciated. I am forever grateful and look forward to being in your presence again really soon.

I would like to extend my gratitude to Daphne Stevenson and the rest of the wonderful ladies of SOMO Book Club. Thank you, ladies for selecting *Dream Weaver the Indigo* as a read and inviting me to your August 2008 book club gathering. I will forever be grateful. I can only hope to be in your presence again someday soon.

To Linda Davis, President of the Illinois chapter of Go on Girl book club, thank you for staying connected and continuing to market my craft at your events. You are truly a blessing. I look forward to being in your presence again really soon.

To my children's principal at Montessori school, Ms. Dilks, thank you for inviting me to your school as well as the book fair at Barnes & Noble to share my experiences as an author. I truly enjoyed being in the presence of the many wonderful fifth, sixth, seventh and eighth graders. It was truly a challenging, as well as rewarding experience.

To the many readers who have read my previous novels, **Dream Weaver the Indigo** and **End of Daze,** I thank you all for your support. I'm a firm believer that reading opens up doors to the dark corners of the mind that have not yet been discovered. I hope my craft continues to illuminate your imagination and intellect while entertaining you well.

To Rachel Lagesse, my energetic source of inspiration, team leader, navigator and most importantly, my supporting comrade in this field of cognitive mental health treatment for juveniles, I couldn't be more blessed to have such a courageous and encouraging team player to stand in the trenches with me during this uphill battle. All the qualities and characteristics I see in myself, I see magnified in you. You are challenging, compassionate, driven, highly energetic and an overachiever which is an amazing gift. You go above and beyond the call of duty to always get it done. I thank you greatly for supporting my craft as a novelist and encouraging me to strive for greatness. If the Marvel comics and the rest of the Super Friends are missing a superwoman, I know where they can find her. Thank you for being extraordinary.

To LaCretia "Cre" Thompson, my colleague, friend and Wonder Woman, thank you for the spiritual warmth and encouraging words that you have often provided in a time of need. Words can't begin to express the level of admiration and respect I have for the energy that embodies you. It is no wonder so many of our colleagues and the children we treat seek you out for advice, comfort and support. You have the gifted ability to make others feel supported. Thank you Wonder Woman for being a wonderful person. It has been an honor to serve as your mentor.

To the rest of my colleagues, James Taylor, Leonard Cooksey, Theo Bey, Dave Samuels, Dave Smith, Dr. Mark Jordan, Mike Chavers, David Hutchinson and many others— thank you all greatly for supporting and acknowledging my efforts, time and work that I have invested into the young people of this population over the years. It is because of you all that I stand where I am in this grand experience. The energy behind the encouraging words you have provided during those tough times keep me humble along this successful path of creativity.

Dr. Tom Kelly and Dr. Antonio Yaniz, thank you both so much for writing the forewords for this novel. I've learned so much about the clinical side of this experience by observing and working closely with the both of you. You are invested in the work that you do and for that I appreciate and respect you greatly. Words can't begin to express my gratitude to you both. The world has so much to learn from you both.

To my children, Wow! You two are incredible. I'm so proud of you both for being creative, challenging, humorous, and oh so inquisitive. I'm so blessed to be a part of your lives not only as your father, but your own personal cheerleader. Remember, never give up on your dreams, the greatest, most powerful gift we've been given in this lifetime is choices and just on the other side of chance is success staring you right in the face. There are no failures only minor setbacks. I luv you both with all the energy that embodies me.

To my Mom and Mr. & Mrs. Randle, thank you for being great parents and grandparents. It takes a whole village to raise a child and the three of you have been that village. I am so grateful for all your support and love.

To my wife, Keisha, the superglue that holds my world together, my queen and my mental and emotional support. Thank you for being my greatest challenge, a challenge that has made be better and stronger. Thank you for giving me a reason to wake up the next day and continue on this journey. Because of your love, I stand strongly where I am today. I especially thank you for being a loving role model and nurturer to our children. Because of that love and nurturing our children have unlimited growth. Love you always.

To my aunts, Hattie and Ruby, thank you for your eagerness and support. The both of you have supported me greatly and I will always and forever be grateful.

To my role models William Smith, Drill Sergeant Carter, Clifton Bey and the late Paul V. Harris, thank you for molding me into the man I am today. Through interacting, listening and observing, I have accepted the love from each of you and chosen to give it back.

www.ingramcontent.com/pod-product-compliance
Lightning Source LLC
Chambersburg PA
CBHW021601280526
45784CB00001BA/456

*9 7 8 1 4 4 0 1 0 4 8 9 3 *